Lead Absorption in Children

Material for this book was adapted from ''Management of Increased Lead Absorption in Children: Clinical, Social, and Environmental Aspects,'' a conference presented by the John F. Kennedy Institute for Handicapped Children and the Johns Hopkins School of Medicine, in Baltimore, Maryland on November 19-20, 1979.

The support of the Office for Maternal and Child Health, Bureau of Community Health Services, Health Services Administration, U.S. Department of Health and Human Services is gratefully acknowledged.

Lead Absorption in Children

Management, Clinical, and
Environmental Aspects

J. Julian Chisolm, Jr.

Project Director
Lead Poisoning Clinic
The John F. Kennedy Institute
Baltimore, Maryland

David M. O'Hara

Acting Director, Social Work
The John F. Kennedy Institute
Baltimore, Maryland

With 46 Illustrations
and 47 Tables

Urban & Schwarzenberg
Baltimore-Munich 1982

Urban & Schwarzenberg, Inc.
7 E. Redwood Street
Baltimore, Maryland 21202
USA

Urban & Schwarzenberg
Pettenkoferstrasse 18
D-8000 München 2
West Germany

Printed in the United States of America

Notice

The Publishers have made a reasonable effort to trace original copyright holders for borrowed material. If they have inadvertently overlooked any, they will be pleased to correct these oversights at the earliest reprint opportunity.

Library of Congress Cataloging in Publication Data

Lead absorption in children.

Proceedings of a conference organized under the auspices and support of the Office of Maternal and Child Health, Bureau of Community Health Services. Includes index.
1. Lead-poisoning in children—Congress.
I. Chisolm, J. Julian, Jr. II. O'Hara, David M. III. United States. Office for Maternal and Child Health. [DNLM: 1. Lead poisoning—In infancy and childhood—Congresses. QV 292 L4302 1979]
RA1231.L4L376   615.9′25688′088054   81-16306
ISBN 0-8067-0331-8   AACR2

Cover design: Roger Maclellan
Compositor: Graphic Arts Composition
Printer: Universal Lithographers
Copy preparation: Deborah Sarsgard
Production and design: John Cronin, Detlev Moos

ISBN 0-8067-0331-8 Baltimore

ISBN 3-541-70331-8 Munich

Contents

Contributors

Paul Burgan, M.D., Ph.D., F.A.A.P.
Mount Washington Pediatric Hospital
Baltimore, Maryland

Michael F. Cataldo, Ph.D.
The John F. Kennedy Institute
Baltimore, Maryland

Lawrence Chadzynski, R.S.
Detroit Department of Health
Herman Kiefer Health Complex
Detroit, Michigan

Evan Charney, M.D.
Sinai Hospital of Baltimore, Inc.
Baltimore, Maryland

J. Julian Chisolm, Jr., M.D.
Lead Poisoning Clinic
The John F. Kennedy Institute
Baltimore, Maryland

Jack W. Finney, M.A.
Pediatric Research Institute
University of Kansas School of
  Medicine
Kansas City, Kansas

Alan Goldberg, Ph.D.
Department of Environmental Health
  Sciences
Division of Toxicology
Johns Hopkins University School of
  Hygiene
Baltimore, Maryland

Robert A. Goyer, M.D.
National Institute of Environmental
  Health Sciences
Research Triangle Park, North
  Carolina

John W. Graef, M.D.
The Children's Medical Center
Boston, Massachusetts

Paul B. Hammond, D.V.M., Ph.D.
Institute of Environmental Health
Kettering Laboratory
University of Cincinnati Medical
  Center
Cincinnati, Ohio

Vernon N. Houk, M.D.
Bureau of State Services
Center for Disease Control
Atlanta, Georgia

Jane S. Lin-Fu, M.D.
Office for Maternal & Child Health
Bureau of Community Health Services
Rockville, Maryland

Nancy A. Madden, Ph.D.
Department of Psychiatry
University of Maryland School of
   Medicine
Baltimore, Maryland

Kathryn R. Mahaffey, Ph.D.
Division of Nutrition, FDA
Cincinnati, Ohio

Christopher Milar, Ph.D.
Division for Disorders of Development
   and Learning
University of North Carolina School of
   Medicine
Chapel Hill, North Carolina

Douglas G. Mitchell, Ph.D.
New York State Department of Health
Division of Laboratories and
   Research
Albany, New York

Hugo W. Moser, M.D.
The John F. Kennedy Institute
Baltimore, Maryland

Paul Mushak, Ph.D.
Division of Environmental Pathology
University of North Carolina School of
   Medicine
Chapel Hill, North Carolina

David M. O'Hara, D.A.S.S.
The John F. Kennedy Institute
Baltimore, Maryland

Lawrence Reiter, Ph.D.
Health Effects Research Laboratory
U.S. Environmental Protection
   Agency
Research Triangle Park, North
   Carolina

Walter J. Rogan, M.D.
National Institute of Environmental
Health Sciences
Research Triangle Park, North
   Carolina

Dennis C. Russo, Ph.D.
Children's Hospital Medical Center
   and Harvard Medical School
Boston, Massachusetts

Estelle Siker, M.D., M.P.H.
Community Health Division
Connecticut State Department of
   Health Services
Hartford, Connecticut

Walter J. Sobolesky, M.S.
Accident Control Section
Department of Public Health
Community Health Services
Philadelphia, Pennsylvania

Preface

Clinical management of the asymptomatic child with increased lead absorption—to be rational—demands an understanding of the many factors which influence the course and outcome of this disorder. The contributions of several disciplines need to be coordinated for effective management. These include: heavy metal metabolism and toxicology; neurotoxicology; nutrition; environmental, behavioral and social sciences; public health; analytical chemistry; environmental hygiene and pediatrics. This volume represents the proceedings of a conference organized under the auspices and support of the Office of Maternal and Child Health, Bureau of Community Health Services, for the purpose of amplifying the clinical dimensions of their various scientific perspectives. Formal papers and discussion focus on the contribution of each discipline to the management of the child with increased lead absorption and are grouped into four sections as follows.

The first part of the book lays the background in metabolism and overall toxicity of lead. As with many environmental toxins, lead has a very slow turnover rate in the body and affects many different organ systems, especially the hematopoietic, nervous and renal systems. Experimental studies have vastly expanded our knowledge of the neurotoxicological effects of lead and reveal that low levels of lead can not only induce maturational delay but also morphological changes that are likely to be permanent. Clinical studies, despite their individual faults, strongly suggest that increased lead absorption without symptoms during early life can lead to subtle disturbances in learning. A lively discussion, including the presentation of some provocative new clinical data, concludes this section.

The second part focuses on environmental, nutritional, behavioral and social factors that can modify the absorption and toxicity of lead in children. The implications of nutritional data suggest that adequate nutrition may play a much greater role in prevention than in treatment. Recent evidence clearly establishes the critical interplay of lead-bearing dust with the normal hand-to-mouth activity of young children as the major route of lead into the body. Not only are dust lead levels high in the home environment of the affected children, but limited data presented at the conference indicate that lead dust is extremely difficult to remove. Clearly, more research in this area is needed. Without the appropriate environmental management, other behavioral and social interventions are of limited efficacy.

Later, the need for close coordination of the health agency, the analytical laboratory, environmental hygiene and clinical disciplines is emphasized. Traditionally, lead has been removed from painted surfaces of dwellings by burning and sanding, which leaves a residue of fine particulate lead in the home. Newer abatement approaches using heat guns and avoidance of sanding give promise of less hazardous abatement procedures in the future. In clinical management, there are clearly similarities between occupational exposure and exposure during childhood. The "dusty trades" have long been recognized as the more hazardous types of occupational exposure to lead. Only recently has the link between dust and increased lead absorption in childhood been appreciated. Treatment of the child, however, is far more difficult than that of the worker. The workman can be removed from his primary source of exposure, the work place, while the child's principal source of exposure is his primary residence, from which he cannot be easily removed. This complicates and limits the effectiveness of treatment in children. Examples are cited of recurrences where exposure in the home persists and, by contrast, improvement often occurs spontaneously, when a new residence is found.

Finally, future clinical directions and research needs are summarized. Walter Rogan provides a comprehensive overview and yet another illustration of idiosyncratic toxicity on the Green Parrot Goat Farm.

The conference and this volume would not have been possible without Dr. Jane S. Lin-Fu, whose longstanding concern for this problem was borne out by her constant support and excellent summation of the history of lead poisoning in children. Thanks must also be given to the participants for their careful attention to the clinical implications of their contributions. Not least is our appreciation for the encouragement of the John F. Kennedy Institute, Hugo W. Moser, M.D., Director.

J. Julian Chisolm, Jr.
David M. O'Hara

Frequently Used Abbreviations

Pb . . . . lead

PbA . . . . air lead (μg Pb/m^3 of air)

PbD . . . . dust lead ppm or μg/unit of exposed surface

PbH . . . . hand lead (μg Pb/hand) as washed off

PbB . . . . blood lead (μg Pb/dl whole blood)

PbU . . . . urine lead (μg Pb/L or μg Pb/24 hr as defined)

PbU-EDTA . chelatable lead, usually expressed as μg Pb excreted/mg CaEDTA administered/24 hr

CaEDTA . . . calcium disodium ethylenediaminetetraacetate

ALAU . . . . . δ-aminolevulinic acid in urine

ALAD . . . . . δ-aminolevulinate dehydratase

FEP . . . . "free" erythrocyte protoporphyrin (μg protoporphyrin/dlerythrocytes)

EP . . . . erythrocyte protoporphyrin (μg protoporphyrin/dl whole blood)

ZnPP . . . . . . zinc protoporphyrin

1. The Evolution of Childhood Lead Poisoning as a Public Health Problem

Jane S. Lin-Fu

Introduction

This paper reviews briefly the evolution of childhood lead poisoning as a public health problem and the metamorphosis in our concept of this illness.

Lead is an extremely useful metal; it has almost become an intrinsic part of our modern way of life. In solder for food cans and electronic equipment, in gasoline, in car and other storage batteries, in craft materials, art works and newsprints, in brasswares, in dinnerwares, crystals and plastics, in caulking and sound-proofing material for buildings, ships and jet planes, in cable covering of intercontinental communication systems, in ammunition, in curtain weights and sinkers for fishing, this metal has found almost endless application since its discovery by man more than 5000 years ago. Following the Industrial Revolution of the 18th century, and particularly since the early 1940's, the use of lead has increased rapidly. Between 1940 and 1977, the consumption of lead in the U.S. almost doubled from 782,000 tons to an estimated 1,505,000 tons (Lead Industries Association, 1978). Between 1935 and 1977, the amount of lead used as a gasoline additive in the U.S. increased six-fold from 37,000 tons to 233,000 tons per year (Lead Industries Association, 1978; National Academy of Science, 1972). It is important to recognize, however, that even though the comfort and convenience of our life style may depend on lead, our life itself does not. Lead plays no physiologic role in the human body.

1

Industrialization, Reproductive Failures and Congenital Lead Poisoning

Our knowledge of lead toxicity dates back at least 2000 years. The problem in children probably first drew attention as congenital lead poisoning in offspring of lead workers following industrialization. In the 18th and 19th centuries, sterility, abortion, stillbirth and premature delivery were common not only in female lead workers, but also among wives of men who worked in lead industries. Infant mortality was extremely high in their offspring, among whom congenital lead poisoning was manifested as low birth weight, convulsions, failure to thrive and mental retardation (Hamilton and Hardy, 1949; Oliver, 1911). Although a high frequency of reproductive failure also occurred in wives of lead workers, removal of women from lead industries in the late 19th century was viewed as some sort of solution to occupational lead poisoning. This is analogous to the removal of children from homes with peeling lead paint without correcting the lead hazard, a practice some still use as a solution to the lead paint poisoning problem today.

With gradual improvement in industrial hygienic standards, congenital lead poisoning became a rarity in the literature. But as late as the period from 1931 to 1940, 853 deaths from lead poisoning in adults were reported in the U.S. (McDonald and Kaplan, 1942). These reported fatality figures tell little of the actual magnitude of the problem of occupational lead poisoning and its byproduct, congenital lead poisoning. The silence of the literature on congenital lead poisoning after the early part of the 20th century should therefore not be equated with the non-existence of the problem.

Discovery of Lead Paint Poisoning in Children

Congenital lead poisoning results from indirect in utero exposure. The prevalence of lead poisoning in children through direct exposure was first observed in Queensland, Australia, in the 1890's (Gibson et al., 1892). The source of lead remained a mystery until 1904, when Gibson traced it to the paint used on railings of verandas and walls in the homes of the children (Gibson, 1904). In the U.S., physicians viewed the Australian experience with some skepticism. In 1914, Thomas and Blackfan of Johns Hopkins published what was perhaps the first case report of lead paint poisoning in the U.S. in a child who chewed the paint off his crib. These authors noted that childhood lead poisoning was uncommon in the U.S. and commented that Australian children "seem peculiarly liable to lead poisoning'' (Thomas and Blackfan, 1914). It was three years later, when Blackfan (1917) reported four other children with convulsions due to lead, that he acknowledged the importance of the Australian studies and noted that lead as a cause of convulsions in children had been largely ignored by U.S. physicians.

A handful of reports of lead meningitis in infants and young children followed Blackfan's paper, but the prevalence of lead poisoning among U.S. children did not gain recognition until 1924, when Ruddock made the important observation that children lived in a ''lead world'' and that pica, or a perverted appetite for non-food items, was important in introducing this toxic element into children's bodies (Ruddock, 1924). In lead paint on houses and furniture, toys, food coloring, food receptacles, cosmetics and even medicinal ointment, lead finds its way into children's mouths. In 1926, McKhann of Boston published the first study of a large series of children with lead poisoning in the U.S. Ingestion of lead paint on cribs and furniture was the cause in most cases (McKhann, 1926).

Lead Poisoning from Burning Battery Casings

In Baltimore, two fatal cases of lead paint poisoning in children attracted the attention of the Health Department in 1931 (Chronology of Lead Poisoning Control, Baltimore, 1931–1971, 1971). This was followed in 1932 by a mass outbreak of lead poisoning primarily involving children which was due to burning of battery casings for fuel in the home (Williams et al., 1933). Similar episodes occurred in Philadelphia, Chicago, Long Island and Detroit (Levinson and Harris, 1936). These outbreaks focused some attention on the problem of lead poisoning in children and its predilection for the poor. In 1935, the Baltimore Health Department's Division of Chemistry began to provide free blood lead tests to physicians and hospitals. This resulted in an increase in the number of diagnosed cases of lead poisoning in children (Kaplan and McDonald, 1942).

Limited Case Findings, 1950's and 1960's

Although the Baltimore Health Department became interested in childhood lead poisoning in the early 1930's, elsewhere health officials gave the problem virtually no attention until the early 1950's. Then a few cities such as New York, Chicago and Philadelphia exerted some effort at case finding and public education. Wherever health workers made such an effort, the number of reported cases invariably increased and the severity of diagnosed cases and fatality rate decreased. But even into the mid-1960's, encephalopathy had often set in before lead poisoning in children was diagnosed. Between 1959 and 1963, physicians at Chicago's Cook County Hospital treated 182 children for lead encephalopathy, of whom 51, or 28%, died (Greengard et al., 1965). Among survivors, sequelae such as convulsions, mental retardation, blindness, cerebral palsy, behavior disorders and learning disabilities were common (Perlstein and Attala, 1966).

That undue exposure of young children to lead reached epidemic proportions is best illustrated by the report of Bradley et al. (1956) of Baltimore. Among 333 children 7 to 60 mos of age from low income areas seen at well-baby clinics and the pediatric outpatient department of the University of Maryland between August 1, 1953, and September 1, 1954, 299 or 90% had blood lead levels of ≥30 μg/100 ml; 86 or 26% had levels of ≥60 μg/100 ml; 197 or 59% had a positive urinary coproporphyrin test; 77 or 23% had positive x-ray evidence of dense metaphyseal lines (so-called "lead lines"). Bradley et al. observed that a blood lead level of ≥50 μg/100 ml was associated with an increase in other findings compatible with the diagnosis of lead poisoning and suggested that this be used as the upper limit of normal. This suggestion went unheeded, and three years later the USPHS recommended that blood lead levels of 60 to 80 μg/100 ml be considered evidence of abnormal lead absorption (National Clearinghouse for Poison Control, 1959).

Epidemiology of Childhood Lead Poisoning, 1950's and 1960's

The epidemiology reports of childhood lead poisoning from different cities from the early 1950's to the middle 1960's yielded a surprisingly uniform pattern (Lin-Fu, 1967).

> Childhood lead poisoning was inextricably related to dilapidated housing where peeling lead paint and broken painted plaster were readily available; the high risk areas or "lead belts" were practically synonymous with large inner city slums. Pica was an important contributing factor. Children 1 to 6 yr, and particularly those 1 to 3 yr, were at greatest risk. Blacks had a higher incidence than whites. Siblings were often affected together. The disease affects children year-round, but symptoms and lead encephalopathy occurred more frequently in the summer. Not unexpectedly, recurrence was the rule unless the lead paint hazard was corrected and, with each recurrence, the prognosis became worse.

Little Action Despite Formidable Data

The formidable data on childhood lead poisoning published in the 1950's and early 1960's troubled surprisingly few health officials, and the public was tragically unaware of their existence. Several factors accounted for this. First, many had mistakenly thought that replacement of the lead pigment by titanium oxide in the early 1940's had solved the lead problem. They failed to realize that millions of houses with layers of old lead paint remained occupied. Others who were aware of the problem considered it an illness inevitable to slum dwelling for which little could be done. The lack of adequate housing codes and the failure to enforce existing ones for financial and other reasons further frustrated interested health workers who knew the return of children to uncorrected housing virtually guaranteed a recurrence. The non-specificity of the symptoms of lead poisoning also confounded the problem, not only for parents, but also for uninformed physicians, since routine physical examination and laboratory studies will not provide an unsuspecting physician with the correct diagnosis (Lin-Fu, 1979).

Acknowledgment of the Problem, Mid-1960's

The turmoil and awakening of social conscience of the mid-1960's brought with it a sudden acknowledgment of the magnitude of childhood lead poisoning. In 1970, the U.S. Surgeon General issued a statement on the disease which shifted the focus from case finding to prevention. He advocated mass screening and early identification of children with evidence of undue lead absorption, defined as a confirmed blood lead level of 40 μg/100 ml or more (Department of Health, Education and Welfare, 1971). That progress cannot be made easily is illustrated by the backward step taken a year later when the American Academy of Pediatrics recommended that the environment of children be investigated only after demonstration of two blood lead levels of $\geq$50 μg/100 ml (American Academy of Pediatrics, 1971).

Mass Screening and Epidemiology, 1970's

The 1971 Lead-Based Paint Poisoning Prevention Act provided, among other things, for Federal assistance through DHEW to help communities carry out screening and treatment programs. Mass screening under the act began in mid-

Table 1. (Risk classifications for asymptomatic children according to various blood lead and erythrocyte protoporphyrin levels. This classification of screening test results is intended to reflect priority for medical evaluation but it is not to be used for diagnostic purposes.) Diagnostic evaluation should be provided more urgently than the classification would otherwise indicate in the following cases: 1) children with any symptoms compatible with lead poisoning: 2) children under 36 mos of age and 3) children whose blood lead and EP values place them in the upper part of a particular class. It must be emphasized the suggested guidelines refer to the interpretation of screening results, but the final diagnosis and disposition rest on a more complete medical and laboratory examination of the individual child. Taken from Preventing Lead Poisoning in Young Children. A Statement by the Center for Disease Control. April 1978.

Test Results	Erythrocyte Protoporphyrin (μg/dl Whole Blood)			
Blood Lead (Mg/dl)	≤49	50-109	110-249	≥250
Not done	I	*	*	*
≤29	I	Ia	Ia	EPP + [†]
30–49	Ib	II	III	III
50–69	‡	III	III	IV
≥70	‡	‡	IV	IV

† Erythropoietic protoporphyria. Although rarely, iron deficiency may cause EP elevations to 300 μg/dl.

* Blood lead necessary to estimate risk.

‡ Combination of results not generally observed in practice; if observed, retest with venous blood immediately.

1971. Data for the first fiscal year are not available. From July 1, 1972, to June 30, 1979, 2,714,413 children were screened; of these, 183,452 or 7% were found to have evidence of undue lead absorption. Beginning in FY 75, children were classified into risk categories according to the Center for Disease Control statement (1978). Of 2,065,112 children screened, 147,334 or 7% had evidence of undue lead absorption. Of these, 103,421 or 5% were in Class II; 35,094 or 2% were in Class III and 8,819 or 0.4% in Class IV. In many cities, more than 15% of the children screened were found to have a lead problem (See Table 1).

With mass screening, it became obvious in the early 1970's that epidemiology of childhood lead poisoning mapped in the 1950's was not quite accurate. Although young children residing in old inner city slums remain at highest risk, the problem of undue exposure to lead extends far beyond the "lead belts" and the poor. It is a nationwide problem which affects rural and middle class children as well. A more careful scrutiny of the lead sources in children's environment reveals that in addition to lead paint and plaster, airborne lead (particularly lead settled in dust and dirt) is an important source of exposure. For children in a polluted environment, even normal hand-to-mouth activities can introduce a toxic amount of lead into their bodies (Lin-Fu, 1973; Sayre et al., 1974). Lead is ubiquitous in our industrialized world; the child, in fact, still lives in a "lead world." Exposure to lead in air, food and drink is inevitable. In addition, lead in paint, dust and dirt and many consumer items that pose little danger to adults, such as colored newsprints and paint on pencils, present a definite hazard to children because of pica and normal hand-to-mouth activities. In the mid-1970's, the danger of occupational lead exposure was found to extend to children of lead workers through exposure to the dust carried home by their parents (Rice et al., 1978). Children living close to lead smelters and processing plants were also found to be unduly exposed to this toxic metal (Landrigan et al., 1975). Sniffing leaded gasoline has also been found to be a source of lead poisoning in children (Seshia et al., 1978).

Lead Paint Versus Other Lead Sources

The discovery of a high lead content of dust and dirt in many urban areas in the early 1970's diverted some attention away from lead paint as the source of poisoning in children. However, experience in the past few years indicates that severe lead poisoning, with rare exceptions, is caused by ingestion of paint or exposure to other high dose sources, such as improperly glazed earthenware. Minor to moderate elevation of blood lead or erythrocyte protoporphyrin may be due to exposure to other lead sources. The lead content of old paint is much higher than that of dust and dirt in polluted areas. It is not unusual for old paint to contain 20 to 30% lead. This compares with a lead content of 20,000 to 30,000 ppm or 2 to 3% in dust and dirt from a highly polluted environment. In El Paso, for example, within 1.6 km of the smelter, the lead content of housedust ranged from 2,800 to 103,750 ppm, with a geometric mean of 22,191 ppm or 2.2% (Landrigan, 1975).

Lead paint, both interior and exterior, poses a danger not only as peeling flakes, but also as a source of housedust and garden soil contamination. It presents a threat to children in dilapidated housing, as well as to middle class children in expensive old houses. Exposure to the lead dust and fumes during renovation of these homes has caused lead poisoning in children (Wolf, 1973); so has burning of painted wood for fuel (DeCastro et al., 1975). The recognition of lead paint as the major source of severe lead poisoning in children does not negate the importance of the other lead sources in contributing to the problem of undue lead absorption in young children. The relative lower lead content of dust and dirt is offset by their small particle size which enhances absorption and by their pervasiveness in the environment of children.

A Change in Clinical
Picture and Focus of Research

Screening and intensive public educational effort in the last decade have reduced dramatically the incidence of lead encephalopathy in children. However, undue lead absorption has continued to be prevalent among children. Since mass screening began in 1971, each year about 6 to 7% of children screened have continued to be found to have undue lead absorption. This is a very troublesome finding, for among these children only 1 out of 7 or 8 meets the current diagnostic criteria for lead poisoning and receives chelation therapy. Do the untreated children escape totally unharmed, or is the damage they sustain too subtle to be detected by routine physical and neurological examination? Studies on the "subclinical" toxic effects of lead have yielded controversial results, but several recent clinical investigations supported by laboratory data are highly suggestive that some "asymptomatic" children may sustain psychoneurological damage at a relatively "low" level of exposure (Needleman et al., 1979; de la Burde and Choate, 1975; Perino and Ernhart, 1974). This subject will be discussed later in this book.

In the last decade, we have witnessed a definite change in the clinical picture of childhood lead poisoning and a shift in the focus of research. From a disease linked to peeling old lead paint encountered only in children from the slums, which often presented as encephalopathy, lead poisoning has become a largely "asymptomatic" state evidenced by an elevated blood lead and/or erythrocyte protoporphyrin level which is associated with multiple sources of exposure affecting a much broader spectrum of children. The focus of both clinical and laboratory investigation has shifted from examining the severe neurological sequelae of lead poisoning such as mental retardation and blindness to exploring subtle psychoneurological deficits and from looking at gross anatomical changes to studying the subcellular effects (Silbergeld and Adler, 1978). The research on lead metabolism has broadened from studying lead absorption and toxicity in isolation to examining the interaction of lead with dietary factors such as iron, calcium, zinc, copper, magnesium, vitamins, fat and amino acids (Mahaffey, 1974). How these factors interplay with lead may hold a key to the puzzling phenomenon of variation in individual susceptibility to lead insult and eventually provide some answers to the troubling issue of "low" level lead toxicity among children.

It is generally conceded that children are more vulnerable to lead injury because of the frequency of pica, hand-to-mouth activity, a greater rate of intestinal absorption and retention and an increased sensitivity of the heme biosynthetic pathway and nervous system to lead insult (Lin-Fu, 1973). But even among children, there is considerable variation; at comparable blood lead levels, some convulse while others are only mildly symptomatic. Some appear to sustain psychoneurological damage at relatively low levels of exposure; others do not.

Conclusion: Lead Poisoning Is Preventable

There remain many missing links in our knowledge about this ubiquitous toxic element. However, it is important to remember that lead poisoning in children is preventable. The dispersion of lead in our environment is man-made and is controllable. A price must be paid for what we have done to our environment in the past. The crucial question is: Shall we pay it in controlling our environment or shall we pay it in terms of the health of thousands of children in our lifetime and millions in generations to come?

References

American Academy of Pediatrics. Committee on Environmental Hazards and Subcommittee on Accidental Poisoning of Committee on Accident Prevention. 1971. Acute and chronic childhood lead poisoning. Pediatrics 47:950–51.

Blackfan, K.D. 1917. Lead poisoning in children with especial reference to lead as a cause of convulsions. Amer J Med Sci 153:877–87.

Bradley, J.E., Powell, A.E., Niermann, W., McGrady, J.R. and Kaplan, E. 1956. The incidence of abnormal blood levels of lead in a metropolitan pediatric clinic. J. Pediatr 49:1–6.

Center for Disease Control. Preventing lead poisoning in young children. A statement by the Center for Disease Control 1978. U.S. DHEW, PHS (Atlanta).

Chronology of Lead Poisoning Control, Baltimore, 1931–1971. Baltimore Health News 1971 48:34–40.

DeCastro, F.J., Lazarra, J. and Rolff, U.T. 1975. Increased lead burden and the energy crisis. Pediatrics 55:573.

de la Burde, B. and Choate, M.S. 1975. Early asymptomatic lead exposure and development at school age. J Pediatr 87:638–42.

Department of Health, Education and Welfare. 1971. Medical aspects of childhood poisoning. U.S. Dept. HEW, Health Services and Mental Health Administration Health Report 86:140–43.

Gibson, J.L. 1904. A plea for painted railings and painted walls of rooms as the source of lead poisoning among Queensland children. Australia Med Gazette 23:149–53.

Gibson, J.L., Love, W., Hardine, D., Bancroft, P. and Turner, A.J. 1892. Note on lead poisoning as observed among children in Brisbane. Trans 3rd Intercolonial Med Congress. Sydney, pp. 76–83.

Greengard, J., Adams, B. and Berman, E. 1965. Acute lead encephalopathy in young children. J Pediatr 66:707–11.

Hamilton, A. and Hardy, H.L. 1949. Industrial Toxicology, 2nd Edition. New York: Paul B. Hoeber, Inc.

Kaplan, E. and McDonald, J.M. 1942. Blood lead determination as a Health Department laboratory service. Am J Public Health 32:481–86.

Landrigan, P.T., Gehlbach, S.H. and Rosenblum, B.F. 1975. Epidemic lead absorption near an ore smelter. The role of particulate lead. N Eng J Med 292:123–29.

Lead Industries Association. 1978. Annual Review 1977. U.S. Lead Industry. New York: LIA Inc.

Levinson, A. and Harris, L.H. 1936. Lead encephalopathy in children. J Pediatr 8:2–15.

Lin-Fu, J.S. 1967. Lead poisoning in children. DHEW Pub No (HSA) 78-5142, revised and reprinted 1970, 1978.

Lin-Fu, J.S. 1973. Vulnerability of children to lead exposure and toxicity. N Eng J Med 289:1229–233, 1289–293.

Lin-Fu, J.S. 1979. Lead poisoning in children. What price shall we pay? Children Today 8:9–13, 36.

Mahaffey, K.R. 1974. Nutritional factors and susceptibility to lead toxicity. Environ Health Perspect 7:107–12.

McDonald, J.M. and Kaplan, E. 1942. Incidence of lead poisoning in the city of Baltimore. JAMA 119:870–72.

McKhann, C.F. 1926. Lead poisoning in children. Am J Dis Child 32:386–92.

National Academy of Science. 1972. Lead: Airborne Lead in Perspective. NAS, Washington, D.C.

National Clearinghouse for Poison Control Center. May 1959. Lead poisoning in children: Diagnostic criteria. U.S. DHEW PHS, Washington, D.C.

Needleman, H.L., Gunnoe, C., Leviton, A., Reed, R., Peresie, H., Maher, C. and Barret, P. 1979. Deficits in psychologic and classroom performance of children with elevated dentine lead levels. N Eng J Med 300:689–95.

Oliver, P. 1911. A lecture on lead poisoning and the race. British Med J 1:1096–98.

Perino, J. and Ernhart, C.B. 1974. The relation of subclinical lead levels to cognitive and sensorimotor impairment in black preschoolers. J Learn Disab 7:26–30.

Perlstein, M.A. and Attala, R. 1966. Neurologic sequelae of plumbism in children. Clin Pediatr 5:292–98.

Rice, C., Fischbein, A., Lilis, R., Sarkozi, L., Kon, S. and Solikoff, I.J. 1978. Lead contamination in the houses of employees of secondary lead smelters. Environ Res 15:375–80.

Ruddock, J.C. 1924. Lead poisoning in children. JAMA 82:1682–684.

Sayre, J.W., Charney, E. and Vostal, J. 1974. House and hand dust as a potential source of childhood lead exposure. Am J Dis Child 127:167–70.

Seshia, S.S., Rajani, K.R., Boeckx, R.L. and Chown, P.N. 1978. The neurological manifestations of chronic inhalation of leaded gasoline. Develop Med Child Neurol 20:323–334.

Silbergeld, E.K. and Adler, H.S. 1978. Subcellular mechanisms of lead neurotoxicity. Brain Res 148:451–67.

Thomas, H.M. and Blackfan, K.D. 1914. Recurrent meningitis due to lead in a child of five years. Am J Dis Child 8:377–80.

Williams, H., Schulze, W.H., Rothcild, H.B., Brown, A.S. and Smith, F.R. 1933. Lead poisoning from the burning of battery casings. JAMA 100:1485–489.

Wolf, M.D. 1973. Lead poisoning from restoration of old homes. JAMA 225:175–76.

2.   Metabolism of Lead

Paul B. Hammond

The term metabolism denotes change, from the Greek "metabole." It is obvious that the term is inappropriate in the case of lead since elements are immutable and, hence not subject to change. A broader definition of metabolism must be considered if anything is to be said about lead which relates to change. One could perhaps describe changes in the nature of lead compounds wherein the metallic ion enters the body as one compound and subsequently becomes transformed to another by active or passive processes. Such changes probably do occur, but not much is known about them. In short, metabolism of lead really is limited to consideration of its movement into, within and out of the body.

Absorption

The major route of lead absorption in children is the gastrointestinal tract. For the forms of lead existing in the normal diet, absorption in children is quite efficient, being on the order of 50%. By contrast, absorption in adults is only approximately 8%. The degree of absorption of other forms of lead is poorly known. Lead in dried paint films is reported to be substantially less well absorbed than lead acetate in 5- to 8-mo-old baboons (Kneip, 1974) and in sexually mature rats (Gage and Litchfield, 1969). By contrast, absorption of lead in ground paint chips is much higher in 21-day-old rats (Table 1).

  Data in animals show that compounds of lead are absorbed from the gastrointestinal tract with varying degrees of efficiency, but it is not known whether this is because the compounds, as such, have a varying ability to pass across the mucosa or whether the enteric environment simply causes varying degrees of solubilization and ionization of the various compounds of lead presented to it. Current dogma has it that the absorption of lead is proportional to the solubility and degree of ionization which occurs in the enteric environment. Variation in lead absorption as related to variation in chemical form is depicted in Table 2. The implication is that the form of lead presented to the pathway of entry simply limits the efficiency of entry and that, once absorbed, all forms of lead behave in identical fashion (Fig. 1). Only one form of lead is known to be absorbed intact and to behave differently from other forms of lead once absorbed. This is the class of alkyl lead compounds added to gasoline, mainly tetraethyllead and tetramethyllead, $(C_2H_5)_4Pb$ and $(CH_3)_4Pb$. These are more efficiently absorbed than other forms of lead, are distributed in the body in a unique manner and cause toxic effects quite unlike those seen with other chemical forms of lead. Childhood exposure to alkyl lead is insignificant, except among those who sniff leaded gasoline for its euphoric effect (Boeckx et al., 1977).

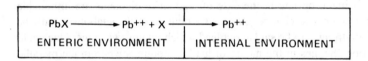

Fig. 1. Lead pathways.

As in man, the absorption of dietary lead by infant rats is very high (50%) and falls rapidly after weaning (Kostial et al., 1971; Forbes and Reina, 1972).

The second major route of absorption obviously is the respiratory system. Virtually nothing is known concerning the peculiarities of infant aerosol physiology. The one obvious difference between infants and adults is the fact that infants inhale far more air in proportion to body weight than adults, owing to their proportionately greater oxygen demand. It follows that pulmonary deposition of inhaled aerosol particles would be correspondingly greater, as would systemic uptake.

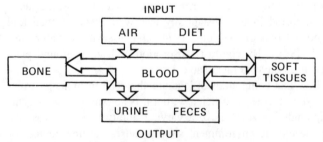

Fig. 2. Lead distribution.

Table 1.   Fecal excretion of lead fed to 21-day-old rats as ground paint chips* (unpublished data from Hammond et al., 1977).

| Day | Rat No. | Fecal Lead Excretion | | Estimated Absorption |
		µg Pb/d	Dose (%)	
0	1	7.6		
1		538.4	49	
2		210.2	19	
3		7.3	<1	
GI content		1.4	<1	
			Total = 68	32%
0	2	1.5		
1		653.0	60	
2		12.8	1	
3		2.9	<1	
GI content		0.6	<1	
			Total = 61	39%

*0.25-1.0 mm mesh size.

Finally, it is likely that percutaneous absorption of lead is essentially insignificant, much as in adults.

Distribution

A single dose of lead, whether by oral administration or by inhalation, is distributed in essentially the same fashion. A three-compartment model of lead distribution is conceptually useful (Fig. 2). The heavy arrow leading from the central compartment (blood) to the bone and the light arrow indicating return from the bone to the blood has profound implications. For the moment, however,

Table 2.   Absorption of lead additives found in paint relative to lead acetate (Barltrop and Meek, 1975).

Lead Compound	Percent Absorption
Control (no lead)	4
Metallic lead (particle size 180–250 µ)	14
Lead chromate	44
Lead octoate	62
Lead naphthenate	64
Lead sulphide	67
Lead tallate	121
Lead carbonate (basic)	164

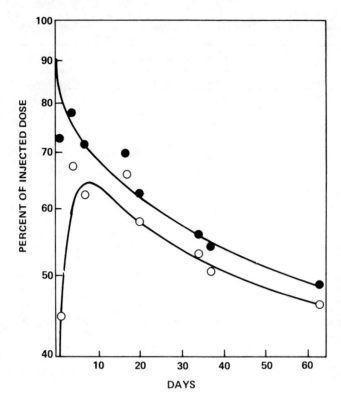

Fig. 3. Fate of a single dose of lead administered to rats. Solid circle, total body Pb; open circle, skeletal Pb (Hammond, 1971. Reprinted with permission of *Toxicology and Applied Pharmacology.*)

it is enough to say that as a result of slow rate of return to the blood, lead accumulates in bone to a much greater extent than in other tissues. This is owing to the inherent affinity of lead for osseous tissue.

The time course for transfer of a single intravenous dose of lead from the central compartment to the other two compartments is illustrated in Figure 3. The data are for rats but are totally consistent with what we know about lead

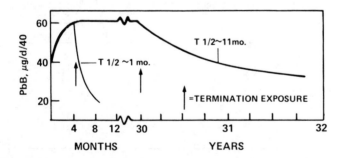

Fig. 4. Effect of duration of high lead exposure on terminal decline of PbB.

metabolism in man except perhaps as to the time scale. These transfers may occur more slowly in man than in rats. In the child, differences among various tissues may also affect transfers.

The most significant implications of the kinetic behavior of lead are its high degree of accumulation upon continued exposure and its slow rate of removal when exposure ceases. Furthermore, the longer the period of high exposure, the slower the rate of removal of lead from the body. This phenomenon is clearly reflected in studies in adults (Fig. 4). The short term disappearance half-time (T½) is from the data of Griffin et al. (1975) and the long term T½ is from the data of Haeger-Aronsen et al. (1974). In the first instance (4 mos of heavy exposure), rapid clearance from the blood is the sum of substantial net transfer into bone superimposed on excretion. In the second instance (after 30 yr of heavy exposure) net transfer into bone is either much smaller or non-existent because the bone pool is probably feeding lead into the circulation at a rate closely matching the transfer of lead from blood into bone (near steady-state conditions). As a result, reduction in PbB is probably largely limited to excretion. The implications of these kinetic principles are numerous. Thus, for example, 1 month in a hazardous environment has much more serious implications than has 1 day in the same environment. Likewise, the need for chelation therapy to reduce circulating lead is much more important following long term exposure than short term exposure.

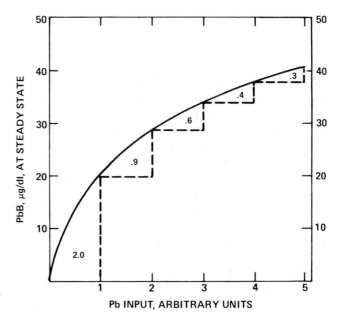

Fig. 5. Relationship between increase in dose and increment in PbB.

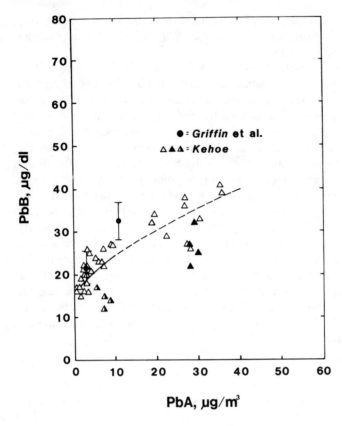

Fig. 6. Increase in PbB associated with increase in PbA in human adults (adapted from Hammond et al., in press).

Since the concentration of lead in the blood is so frequently used as an index of lead exposure, it is important to consider its relationship to rate of input. The source is not important in this context. What is important is the fact that the relationship is non-linear. As the dose increases, the incremental rise in PbB becomes progressively smaller (Fig. 5). Real-life data amply support the validity of the generalization. The assemblage of data for air lead (PbA) versus PbB, illustrated in Figure 6, is composed of data points from experimental studies in which PbA was measured with personal monitors along with PbB. This decreasing incremental rise in PbB is even more dramatically illustrated when one plots the ratio of PbB/PbA against increasing PbA (Fig. 7). A similar curvilinear relationship exists in the case of the impact of lead in water on PbB (Moore et al., 1977).

Perhaps the most significant implication is in regard to the effect on PbB of removing lead from the child's internal environment (chelation) or external environment (clean-up). The higher the PbB, the greater the amount of reduction in intake necessary to reduce PbB by a particular increment, e.g., 10 μg/dl.

Table 3.   No detected effect levels in terms of PbB (µg of lead per 100 ml of blood) (WHO, 1977).

No Detected Effect Level	Effect	Population
<10	Erythrocyte ALAD inhibition	Adults, children
20–25	FEP	Children
20–30	FEP	Adult, female
25–35	FEP	Adult, male
30–40	Erythrocyte ATPase inhibition	General
40	ALA excretion in urine	Adults, children
40	CP excretion in urine	Adults
40	Anaemia	Children
40–50	Peripheral neuropathy	Adults
50	Anaemia	Adults
50–60	Minimal brain dysfunction	Children
60–70	Minimal brain dysfunction	Adults
60–70	Encephalopathy	Children
>80	Encephalopathy	Adults

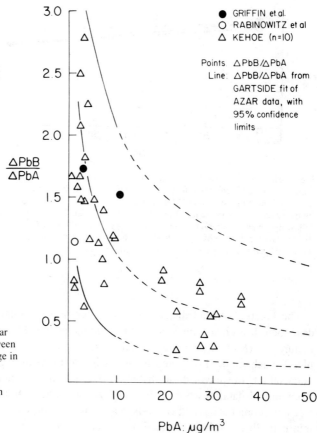

Fig. 7. Inverse curvilinear relationship in man between air lead (PbA) and change in blood lead/air lead ratio (ΔPbB/ΔPbA) (adapted from Hammond et al., in press. Reprinted with permission of *Food and Cosmetics Toxicology*.)

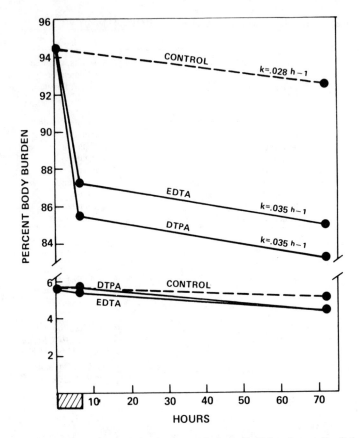

Fig. 8. The effects of chelation therapy on the loss of lead from bone and soft tissues of the rat. The upper portion represents the effect of chelation therapy on the lead in bone and the lower portion the effect on lead in the soft tissues. Both EDTA and DTPA were infused over the initial 6 hr as depicted by the hatched block in the lower left corner of the graph. Treatments were initiated 17 days following the administration of lead, 7 mg Pb/kg with 100–400 μCi^{210}Pb/kg. The rate constant k is the constant for the rate of loss of lead from bone in the control animals and in the treated animals during the period following termination of drug infusion.

The kinetics of lead distribution and excretion in children is not very well described. It is clear, however, that infant rats retain lead much more avidly than mature rats (Momcilovic and Kostial, 1975). Moreover, lead is cleared from the blood much more slowly and localizes in the brain to a greater degree in the neonatal rat. In spite of these striking differences in lead metabolism, as inferred from animal data, newborn babies and young children living in relatively lead-free environments have PbB levels very similar to those of adults. Moreover, the minimal PbB levels associated with specific toxic effects of lead are only

somewhat lower in young children than in adults, as summarized in the World Health Organization 1977 report on lead (Table 3).

It should be mentioned in passing that chelation therapy exerts its major lead-mobilizing action on the exchangeable pool of lead in bone. Thus, in rats, a standard infusion of EDTA removes eight times as much lead from the bone pool as from the soft tissue pool (Fig. 8) (Hammond, 1971). The same is true of other major chelating agents used in the treatment of lead poisoning, d-penicillamine and British Anti-Lewisite (BAL). Again, for purposes of comparing adults to infants, it is necessary to fall back on rat data. In this species, at least, chelation therapy removes lead far more efficiently in adults than in infants (Jugo et al., 1975).

Summary of Lead Metabolism

The metabolism of lead in children and adults is compared. Inorganic forms of lead are of major concern. These are much more efficiently absorbed from the gastrointestinal tract in children than adults ($\sim$50% versus $\sim$8%). Animal studies suggest that lead also is excreted more rapidly in adults than in the very young, both spontaneously and under the influence of chelating agents, e.g., EDTA. Yet, in spite of greater absorption and slower excretion, normal blood concentrations in adults and children are very similar and threshold blood lead concentrations for a variety of toxic effects are only moderately lower in children than in adults.

References

Barltrop, D. and Meek, F. 1975. Postgrad Med J 51:805.

Boeckx, R.L., Posti, B. and Coodin, F.J. 1977. Pediatrics 60:140.

Gage, J.C. and Litchfield, M.H. 1969. J Oil Chem Assn 52:236.

Griffin, T.B., Coulston, F., Wills, H., Russell, J.C. and Knelson, J.H. 1975. Environmental Quality and Safety, Supplement volume II: Lead, Ed. T.B. Griffin and J.H. Knelson., G. Theime, Stuttgart.

Haeger-Aronsen, B., Abdulla, M. and Fristedt, B.J. 1974. Arch Environ Hlth 29:150.

Hammond, P.B. 1971. Toxicol Appl Pharmacol 18:296.

Hammond, P.B., Clark, C.S., Gartside, P., Berger, O. and Michael, L.W. 1977. Final report to NSF-RANN. Grant 77-22186.

Hammond, P.B., Clark, C.S., Gartside, P.S., Berger, O., Walker, A. and Michael, L. W. 1980. Fecal lead excretion in young children as related to sources of lead in their environments. Int Arch Occup Environ Health 46:191-202.

Hammond, P.B., O'Flaherty, E.J. and Gartside, P.S. The impact of air lead on blood lead. A critique of the recent literature. Food and Cosmetics Toxicology, in press.

Jugo, A., Maljkovic, T. and Kostial, K. 1975. Environ Res 10:271.

Kehoe, R.A. 1979. Oral and Inhalation Lead Exposures in Human Subjects (Kehoe Balance Experiments), Lead Industries Assn. Inc. (assembled by S.B. Gross).

Kneip, T. 1974. Lead Toxicity Studies in Infant Baboons. Final report to the Consumer Product Safety Commission. Contract CPSC-C-74-153.

Momcilovic, B. and Kostial, K. 1975. Environ Res 10:271.

Moore, M.R., Meredith, P.A., Campbell, B.C. and Goldberg, A. 1977. Lancet II:661.

Rabinowitz, M.B. 1974. Lead contamination of the biosphere by human activity. A stable isotope study. Ph.D. Thesis, University of California at Los Angeles.

World Health Organization. 1977. Environmental Health Criteria 3. Lead. World Health Organization, Geneva.

3. Lead Toxicity

Robert A. Goyer

Introduction

In this presentation, an overview on the various effects of lead on the different organ systems will be provided, along with clinical signs and symptoms with pathological effects, at least to the degree that we know them. We will attempt to relate dose of lead to these particular effects, to the extent that information is available.

Concepts of Dose

In terms of dose and exposure to lead, the major concern of physicians is, the no-effect level of lead, or the level below which no adverse health effect occurs. Of all the questions asked about lead, this is probably the most difficult to answer. Conceptually, it seems simple and straight forward. However, it is now possible to identify biochemical effects of lead in persons in the general population, presumably in the absence of any adverse health effect. Determining the level at which these biochemical effects should be regarded as toxic or pathologic is probably the greatest challenge in research on the biologic effects of lead today. Since the no-effect level of lead is in some instances difficult to ascertain, two other approaches have been attempted in order to provide specific guidance in the interpretation of dose-effect relationships for lead. However, the specific data for both of these expressions are quite limited.

The dose-effect relationship is really the intensity of a specific effect in an individual at a particular dose. This is the result that a physician gets in a

21

laboratory test and relates to other laboratory data or clinical features. For example, a blood lead level of 60 μg/dl in a child with 9 g of hemoglobin/dl of blood is a specific dose-effect relationship. With a large number of determinations, such as many observations by pediatricians of doses of lead associated with various hemoglobin levels, dose-response relationships and the relative frequency of occurrence of specific effects can be determined. As a further example of dose-population response rates, it has been determined that about 5% of adults will have a greater than 40% inhibition of δ-aminolevulinic acid dehydratase (ALA-D) at a blood lead level of 20 μg/dl. These examples serve to introduce two types of dose relationships, dose-effect in individuals and population dose-response rates as determined in groups.

I would like to make some comments about qualifying terms that have been applied to effects of lead because they have certain clinical implications. The term subclinical, in contrast to clinical, is used to describe measurable effects of lead, mostly biochemical effects and functional effects on the central nervous system, that are not obvious clinically. The terms acute and chronic apply to clinical toxicity; they are not always related to acuteness or chronicity of exposure, but rather apply to the abruptness of onset of symptoms. If the effect is persistent or irreversible, then the term chronic may be applied. For instance, a child who is thought to be well by his family who suddenly develops central nervous system effects is usually referred to as having acute toxicity, even though the exposure to lead may antecede his clinical features by weeks or months. On the other hand, chronic lead poisoning from long term exposure may result in some irreversible effect such as decreased intelligence or motor function without any symptoms that a clinician would regard as acute. Another example of how the term chronic is applied in lead poisoning is illustrated by the renal disease that a lead worker may experience. Here there is long term heavy exposure with no obvious acute clinical symptoms followed by symptoms of kidney disease. This is referred to as chronic lead nephropathy.

We now have also the term ''low level lead exposure.'' This usually refers to the effect resulting from long term lead doses that might be quite tolerable for a few days; however, for the longer period the dose is cumulative, so that clinical toxicity occurs. It is often difficult to identify the source of long term low level exposure; it may be from multiple environmental sources. Lead toxicity is seldom acute in the sense that we use the term for other clinical disorders. The adverse effects of lead reflect the progressive accumulation of excessive amounts of lead.

Here we will review the effects of lead in organ systems, particularly the hematopoietic system, the nervous system and the renal system, including some comments about fetal-maternal relationships. There are also effects of lead on other organ systems that may be important (i.e., thyroid, myocardium), but they have not been studied to the same degree and they are not as impressive clinically.

Measurement of Dose of Lead

Some comments about the measurement of the dose of lead are in order. Theoretically, the most informative or meaningful measure of dose is the concentration of lead in the organ in which the symptoms originate. This is referred to as the critical organ concentration. In the absence of a sample of tissue or a biopsy specimen, we must rely on lead content of biologic fluids. The choices are generally urine or blood, and it is generally agreed that lead in blood is the best measure of dose. We must also recognize that blood lead really reflects recent exposure to lead; occasionally when blood lead is unexpectedly low, it may simply mean that the blood lead was much higher at some earlier time. However, this implies that there may not be a constant relationship between blood lead and organ concentration. Another problem with blood lead is that it may be influenced by several extraneous factors, not the least of which is variation in analytical methodology.

Some fraction of any lead that is absorbed is retained. The major depository is bone. One of the most effective ways to measure body burden of lead was described by Chisolm and Harrison in 1956. They first correlated the urinary excretion of lead following the administration of a standard dose of calcium disodium ethylenediamine tetraacetate (CaEDTA) with biochemical effects of lead on heme synthesis, as have many others since that time. They proposed that increases in the excretion of lead in urine following a standardized dose will reflect increases in the "metabolically active" or toxic fraction of the total body lead burden. Another effort to estimate the total body exposure is by measuring lead in hair. Hair grows about 1 cm a month and, by measuring the lead content of hair segmentally, one gets a profile of past exposure depending on the length of the hair. Studies on lead in hair have met with variable success, the major problem has been laboratory procedure. It is a very tedious job to cut the hair in segments, wash it properly and make all the analyses.

Hematopoietic Effects of Lead

Probably the most sensitive parameters of biologic effects of lead are in the hematopoietic system. The clinical end point is anemia, which seems to occur at a much lower lead level in children than it does in adults. This may reflect that anemia in the child is influenced by a variety of other nutritional factors that may not be as evident in adults. The characteristics of lead-induced anemia are that it is microcytic and morphologically not different from iron deficiency anemia. And, of course, the anemia of lead poisoning is often accompanied by iron deficiency. Basophilic stippling is not very useful in determining exposure to lead. It is nonspecific. It occurs usually at high dose levels with some microcytosis or even some measurable anemia. This parameter is not very useful today and there are no dose-response data of which I am aware.

The anemia of lead probably has three bases. Red blood cell survival is decreased. There is impairment of globin synthesis and there is also some inhibition of heme synthesis. Much is known about inhibition of heme synthesis by lead, because there are biochemical markers of the effects that are easily measurable. The rate-limiting step is not known (that is, whether the degree of anemia is more importantly related to decrease in red cell survival, globin synthesis or inhibition of heme synthesis). However, measurements of various enzymes and intermediates in heme synthesis have been found to be very useful clinically.

Figure 1 shows essential steps in heme synthesis. At least three steps in heme synthesis may be affected by lead. ALA-D is probably the enzyme in the heme pathway that is most sensitive to lead. Inhibition of this enzyme results in a block in utilization of ALA and in subsequent decline in heme synthesis. Secondly, in the scheme of negative feedback control of heme synthesis, ALA synthetase

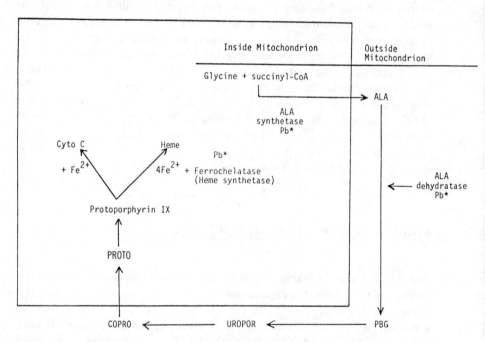

Fig. 1. Scheme of heme synthesis showing sites where lead has an effect. PGB, porphobilinogen; UROPOR, Uroporphyrinogen; COPRO, coproporphyrinogen; PROTO, protophorphyrinogen; CoA, coenzyme A; ALA, δ-aminolevulinic acid; Pb* site for Pb effect.

activity is derepressed, which results in increased activity of the enzyme and increased synthesis of ALA.

A third abnormality of heme synthesis in lead intoxication is inhibition of the enzyme ferrochelatase. Ferrochelatase catalyzes the incorporation of the ferrous iron into the porphyrin ring structure. Bessis and Jensen (1965) have shown that iron in the form of ferritin and ferruginous micelles may accumulate in mitochondria of bone marrow reticulocytes from lead-poisoned rats.

Other steps in the biosynthetic pathway of heme may also be abnormal in lead toxicity, but the evidence for this is incomplete. Increase in urinary excretion of coproporphyrin (CP), the degradative product of coproporphyrinogen (COPRO), is a sensitive reflection of lead toxicity. Metabolism of porphobilinogen (PGB) to coproporphyrinogen proceeds unimpaired, but increased urinary excretion of both of these metabolites does occur in lead poisoning and the mechanism is not understood. It has been shown (Piper and Tephly, 1974) that lead inhibits erythrocytic uroporphyrinogen synthetase but has little effect on the hepatic enzyme. These results suggest that the source of PBG excretion following lead poisoning may be from red blood cells. ALA-D is an extramitochondrial enzyme and later steps in heme synthesis are intramitochondrial. Incorporation of coproporphyrinogen into the mitochondrial matrix might be impaired in the presence of altered inner membrane permeability and reduction in oxidation and phosphorylation (Haeger-Aronsen et al., 1968). Whether the increase in urinary COPRO that occurs in lead poisoning represents a nonspecific alteration in mitochondrial membranes or reflects a more specific effect of lead on the intramitochondrial enzyme coproporphyrinogenase is not known.

Interference of lead in heme synthesis also results in increase in so-called "free erythrocyte protoporphyrin" (FEP) in blood. It has been shown that FEP is not really "free," but is the metalloporphyrin zinc protoporphyrin IX (ZnPP) (Lamola and Yamane, 1974). The inhibition of ferrochelatase by lead prevents the introduction of iron into protoporphyrin IX to form heme. Both in iron deficiency and lead poisoning, the porphyrin chelates Zn non-enzymatically to form ZnPP which, in turn, becomes incorporated into hemoglobin. ZnPP containing hemoglobin has a much lower oxygen carrying capacity than Fe-containing hemoglobin but is usually present in only small amounts (less than 1% of hemoglobin) even in severe lead poisoning. Nevertheless, it is firmly bound within heme and persists there for the life span of the red blood cell, about 120 days (Blumberg et al., 1977). Because ZnPP-containing globin fluoresces when excited, it may be measured fluoremetrically and provides a very sensitive indicator of lead exposure.

Figure 2 illustrates population dose-response relationships between various parameters of heme synthesis. Each curve represents the plotting of a number of observations. Between a blood lead of 20 to 30 µg/dl, a 40% decrease in ALA-D activity might be expected in from 20 to 70% of the population. If the numbers of observations are increased, the tail of the curve is lengthened in both directions

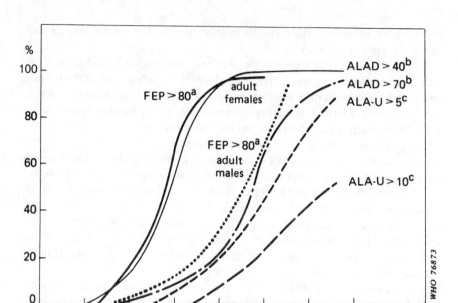

Fig. 2. Dose response relationships for some effects of lead; a, μg/dl of erythrocytes; b, inhibition, c, mg/liter (from WHO, Environmental Health Criteria, Lead, 1977).

so that the most and least sensitive members of the population are identified. The middle of the curve is relatively stable; this is a useful concept to determine how a particular patient relates to people in the general population. If a child with a blood lead of 40 μg/dl has a normal ALA-D, you might conclude that something was wrong with the blood lead or that this child was unusually resistant to the effect of lead on this aspect of heme synthesis.

Central Nervous System Effects

The central nervous system effects of lead may occur over a wide range of blood lead levels. Historically, the only recognized effect of lead on the central nervous system has been acute lead encephalopathy, but now it is known that there are more subtle effects at low blood lead levels as well. Acute encephalopathy is unlikely unless blood lead levels exceed 80 to 100 μg/dl. At 80 μg/dl, severe but not life-threatening effects on the central nervous system can be expected in most children. There may be progression to intellectual dullness and reduced consciousness and eventually seizures, coma and perhaps death. Thirty years ago a child was not recognized as having central nervous system effects of lead until these symptoms occurred. Fortunately, these effects are uncommon today.

It has been learned from autopsy studies that there are two types of morphologic effects in the central nervous system with lead encephalopathy. There is almost always severe cerebral edema which seems to have as its basis some injury to capillaries. Secondly, there is a direct toxic effect on neurons, including actual loss of neurons in particular areas of the brain where neurons are most concentrated (in gray matter, generally thalamus, hypothalamus, and basal ganglia). Associated with the loss of neurons is an increase in glial cells. The gliosis and loss of neurons probably represent the duration as well as severity of lead exposure. Cerebral edema may be regarded as reversible, whereas loss of neurons and gliosis is irreversible. The irreversibility of these effects of lead on the nervous system is documented in long term follow-up studies of children who survived this experience. A certain percentage of these children have seizures, mental retardation and behavioral changes.

Recent studies suggest that sub-clinical or difficult to detect effects on central nervous function, particularly intelligence and behavioral activity, are present in children with blood lead levels over 40 μg/dl. Pueschel and coworkers (1972) conducted a comprehensive study of 58 asymptomatic children with increased body burden of lead as demonstrated by blood lead over 50 μg/dl or urinary lead exceeding 500 μg/μ 24 hr following a CaEDTA-provocative test. Mild central nervous system symptoms such as clumsiness and irritability were observed in one third of the 59 children. Minor neurological dysfunction and various forms of motor impairment were detected by more elaborate testing in 22 to 27% of the children tested. Chelation therapy was given and measures were taken to improve their home environment. Eighteen months later a significant improvement in some areas of intellectual performance was observed.

David and coworkers (1972) have found that after a single dose of a chelating agent lead levels in urine were more increased in hyperactive than in non-hyperactive children. This implies a role for raised lead levels in hyperactivity. Moreover, over one-half of the hyperactive children (28 of 54) had blood lead levels between 25 and 65 μg/dl. These workers argue that any blood lead elevation over 24.5 μg/dl is dangerous and may produce central nervous system effects. In addition, de la Burdè and Choate (1975) showed that a group of 70 selected 4-yr-old children asymptomatic for lead poisoning but with elevated blood lead levels (mean 58 μg/dl, range 40 to 100 μg/dl) or a lead level of at least 30 μg/dl with positive radiographic findings of lead lines in long bones and/or metallic densities in the intestines had deficits in fine motor function and behavior. Follow-up of 67 of these children 3 years later (at 7 yr of age) showed continued deficits in behavior and fine motor coordination, as well as deficits in global IQ (de la Burdè and Choate, 1975). Each of these studies thus suggests that when blood lead levels exceed 40 μg/dl adverse health effects may occur, but no correlation is yet possible between minimal effects for a particular level of lead exposure and/or blood lead concentration.

A large number of experimental studies have investigated the effects of prenatal and neonatal lead exposure on central nervous system development and behavior. These studies have variable results, forming a spectrum that includes delayed nervous system development, deficits in visual motor function, abnormal social and aggressive behavior, hyperactivity and hypoactivity, as well as no changes in activity (Damstra, 1977).

Peripheral Nervous System Effects

Peripheral neuropathy is a classical manifestation of lead toxicity, particularly in adults with excessive occupational exposure. In an early clinical study of neuropathy in lead-poisoned adults, nearly two-thirds of 55 patients were found to have some degree of muscle weakness and almost one-half had·wrist drop (Thomas, 1904).

Children may also develop peripheral neuropathy with chronic lead poisoning. It is said that wrist drop is the most common manifestation of lead neuropathy in adults, while foot drop and generalized weakness are more common in children (Seto and Freeman, 1964).

Electrophysiologic measurements of nerve conduction on men with occupational exposure to lead often show a significant decrease in nerve impulse amplitude when compared to a non-lead exposed control group (Fullerton and Harrison, 1969; Catton et al., 1970). However, more recently Seppalainen and coworkers (1975) demonstrated reduction in nerve conduction velocities and electromyographic deficits in lead workers whose blood lead levels were between 50 and 70 μg/dl.

Effects of Lead on Reproduction

Severe lead intoxication has long been associated with sterility, abortion, stillbirths and neonatal deaths in humans (Nishimura, 1964; Gillet, 1955; Potter, 1961), but evidence that lead poisoning affects birth rate or causes injury to the fetus is not conclusive. Studies with rabbits, guinea pigs and rats indicate that ingestion of lead by either parent may have an effect on reproductive performance. Both size and number of offspring are reduced (Cole and Bachhuber, 1914; Weller, 1951; Morris et al., 1938; Dalldorf and Williams, 1945). Stowe and Goyer (1971) have shown that ingestion of lead by offspring (F_1 generation) of lead-burdened parents results in decreased reproductive fitness. Both paternal and maternal effects were recognized.

Paternal ingestion of lead appears to result in retardation of embryonic growth of the offspring and in a reduction in the number of weaned pups per litter. These observations may indicate a defect in the spermatozoa of lead-intoxicated males which fertilize the normal ova. No morphological or functional (motility) differences were found between sperm from control and lead-fed parents.

The maternal effects of lead are exhibited by reduced litter size, retardation of fetal development and impaired postnatal survival. These effects may be classified as gametotoxic, intrauterine and extrauterine. The combined male and female effects of lead toxicity on overall reproductive ability were greater when both parents had increased lead burdens, which suggests different effects in both parents as well as additive effects. The ovaries of lead-burdened mothers show a reduced number of developing follicles. Similar morphological changes have been observed in ovaries of rhesus monkeys with lead intoxication (Vermande-Van Eck and Meigs, 1960). The offspring in these experiments did not have any congenital malformations.

Selective teratological damage occurs in the caudal region of offspring of Golden Hamsters only when lead salts are injected on the 8th day of gestation (Ferm and Carpenter, 1967). Lead has been shown to be teratogenic to chick embryos, but in these experiments there was direct injection of high doses of lead to the embryos at 2 days of age.

There have been few well-documented reports on reproductive effects of lead in humans. Lead does cross the human placenta as early as the 12th week of gestation (Barltrop, 1969). Cord-blood content of lead shows a high correlation with maternal-blood samples, suggesting that infants are exposed in utero to blood lead levels equivalent to those of the mother (Gershanik et al., 1974).

There are, however, no conclusive reports that lead is teratogenic in man, although there is still much uncertainty with regard to subtle prenatal effects and the possibility that the fetus may be more susceptible than the mother to the effects of a particular level of lead exposure.

A number of as yet inconclusive reports have been published on the chromosomal effects of excessive exposure to lead. Muro and Goyer (1969) found an increased number of gap-break type aberrations in mice receiving a diet containing 1% lead acetate. Similar gap-break types are also found in lead workers with blood lead levels ranging from 62 to 88 μ/100 g. In addition, a variety of nonspecific changes in chromosome morphology was also present, such as adhesions and spiralizing defects. Tetraploid mitoses and the mitotic index were also increased in the workers. Moreover, the percentage of abnormal mitoses correlated very well with urinary ALA excretion (Schwanitz et al., 1970). Deknudt et al. (1973) found chromosomal damage in 14 male workers with clinically evident lead poisoning. Forni and Secchi (1973) showed that the rates of chromatidal changes were higher in 65 workers with pre-clinical and clinical signs of lead poisoning, but were not increased in workers with only a past history of lead poisoning.

On the other hand, O'Riordan and Evans (1974) did not find any significant increases in chromosomal damage in workers in a ship-breaking yard, although some workers had blood lead levels as high as 120 µg/dl.

Renal Effects of Lead

Early or Reversible Lead Nephropathy

Acute effects of lead on the kidney were distinguished from lead-induced chronic nephropathy more than 50 years ago by the English toxicologist Thomas Oliver (1914). Acute renal effects of lead are seen in persons dying of acute lead poisoning or suffering from lead-induced anemia and/or encephalopathy and are usually restricted to nonspecific degenerative changes in renal tubular lining cells, usually causing cloudy swelling and some degree of cellular necrosis. Cells of the proximal convoluted tubules are most severely affected.

Regarding functional affects, Wilson and coworkers first reported hypoaminoaciduria in the presence of normal plasma amino acids in 1953. Dysfunction of proximal renal tubules (Fanconi's syndrome), as manifested by aminoaciduria, glycosuria, and hyperphosphaturia in the presence of hypophosphatemia and rickets was first noted in acute lead poisoning by Chisolm and coworkers (1955). Subsequently, Chisolm (1962) found the Fanconi syndrome in 9 of 23 children with acute lead encephalopathy. Following treatment, all abnormal findings, including rickets, reverted to normal in these children.

Intranuclear inclusion bodies in renal tubular lining cells occur early in the course of excessive exposure to lead (Fig. 3) and ultrastructural studies of renal biopsies of lead workmen, as well as experimental animals, show bizarre mitochondrial alterations, as described. The inclusion bodies are lead protein complexes and sequester intracellular lead.

There is little evidence that the glomerulus is directly affected by excessive exposure to lead, at least in the early stages of lead nephropathy. A recent report suggests that a lowered glomerular filtration rate occurs in subclinical occupational exposure to lead (Wedeen et al., 1975), but this is difficult to reconcile with the only slightly reduced glomerular function found in workmen with more than 10 years of heavy lead exposure and symptoms of lead toxicity (Cramer et al., 1974).

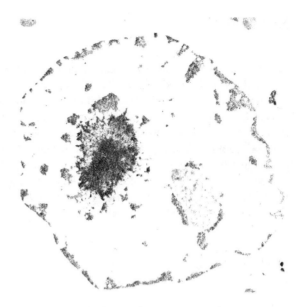

Fig. 3. Nucleus of proximal renal tubular lining cell containing large dense inclusion body characterized by fibrillary margins. The lead-induced inclusion body is separate from the nucleolus.

Renal tubular dysfunction (Fanconi syndrome) disappears after treatment with chelating agents along with clinical remission of other symptoms of lead toxicity (Chisolm, 1962, 1968). It has also been shown experimentally that the nuclear inclusion bodies are removed with chelation therapy and mitochondrial ultra-structure is restored to normal (Goyer and Wilson, 1975). For these reasons it is believed that the early effects of lead on the kidney are reversible.

Chronic or Irreversible Lead Nephropathy

Men with continued occupational exposure to lead and experimental animals exposed to long term intake of lead salts develop toxic or interstitial nephropathy that is not reversible. Also, recent study of mortality patterns in men who worked in lead production facilities and battery plants has shown a greater than expected incidence of "unspecified nephritis or renal sclerosis" (Cooper and Gaffey, 1975).

The morphological features of chronic lead nephropathy consist of a progres-sive increase in interstitial fibrosis between tubules in the renal cortex with eventual loss of functional tubules (Goyer, 1971). There are no specific tests of renal function that are predictive of transition from early or reversible lead nephropathy to irreversible changes apart from renal biopsy and morphological studies.

Summary

This brief review has related clinical manifestations and pathological effects of lead toxicity with blood lead levels, which are the most convenient measure of lead dose. Erythrocyte ALA-D inhibition is the most sensitive measure of lead effect. The no-effect level may be as low as 10 μg/dl of blood. FEP elevation may occur in children with blood lead levels between 20 to 25 μg Pb/dl of blood, whereas anemia might not occur until blood lead is ⩾40 μg/dl of blood.

Minimal brain dysfunction and peripheral neuropathy are not easily demonstrated in children with blood lead levels below 40 μg/dl Pb whole blood, but the no-effect level may not be known because of the lack of sensitive tools for measuring nervous system function.

References

Barltrop, D. 1969. Transfer of lead to the human foetus. In Mineral Metabolism in Paediatrics (D. Barltrop and W.L. Burland, eds.), p. 139. Blackwell, Oxford.

Bessis, M.D. and Jensen, W.N. 1965. Sideroblastic anemia, mitochondria and erythroblastic iron. Brit J Haematol 11:49–51.

Blumberg, W.E., Eisenger, J., Lamola, A.A. and Zuckerman, D.M. 1977. Zinc protoporphyrin level in blood determined by a portable hematofluorometer: A screening device for lead poisoning. J Lab Clin Med 89:712–723.

Catton, M.J., Harrison, M.J.G., Fullerton, P.M. and Kazantzis, G. 1970. Subclinical neuropathy in lead workers. Brit Med J 2:80–82.

Chisolm, J.J., Jr. 1962. Aminoaciduria as a manifestation of renal tubular injury in lead intoxication and a comparison with patterns of aminoaciduria seen in other diseases. J Pediat 60:1–17.

Chisolm, J.J., Jr. 1968. The use of chelating agents in the treatment of acute and chronic lead intoxication in childhood. J Pediat 73:1–38.

Chisolm, J.J., Jr., Harrison, H.C., Eberlein, W.R. and Harrison, H.E. 1955. Amino-aciduria, hypophosphatemia, and rickets in lead poisoning. Study of a case. Am J Dis Child 89:159–168.

Chisolm, J.J., Jr. and Harrison, H.E. 1956. Quantitative urinary coproporphyrin excretion and its relation to edathamil calcium disodium administration in children with acute lead intoxication. J Clin Invest 35:1131–1138.

Cole, L.J. and Bachhuber, L.J. 1914. The effect of lead on the germ cells of the male rabbit and fowl as indicated by their progeny. Proc Soc Exp Biol Med 12:24–31.

Cooper, W.C. and Gaffey, W.R. 1975. Mortality of lead workers. J Occup Med 17:100–107.

Cramer, K., Goyer, R.A., Jagenburg, R. and Wilson, M.H. 1974. Renal ultrastructure, renal function, and parameters of lead toxicity in workers with different period of lead exposure. Brit J Ind Med 31:113–127.

Dalldorf, G. and Williams, R.R. 1945. Impairment of reproduction in rats by ingestion of lead. Science 102:668–670.

Damstra, Terri 1977. Toxicological properties of lead. Environ Health Perspect 19:297–307.

David, O.J., Clark, J. and Voeller, K. 1972. Lead and hyperactivity. Lancet 2:900–903.

Deknudt, G.H., Leonard, A. and Ivanov, B. 1973. Chromosome aberrations observed in male workers occupationally exposed to lead. Environ Physiol Biochem 3:132–138.

de la Burdè, B. and Choate, M.S. 1975. Does asymptomatic lead exposure in children have latent sequelae? J Pediatr 81:1088–1091.

Ferm, V.H. and Carpenter, S.J. 1967. Developmental malformations resulting from the administration of lead salts. Exp Mol Pathol 7:208–213.

Forni, A. and Secchi, G.C. 1973. Chromosome changes in preclinical and clinical lead poisoning and correlation with biochemical findings. In Proc Intern Symp Environ Health Aspects of Lead, Amsterdam, October 2-6, 1972, p. 473.

Fullerton, P.M. and Harrison, M.J. 1969. Subclinical lead neuropathy in man. Electroencephalog Clin Neurophysiol 27:718–719.

Gershanik, J.J., Brooks, G.G. and Little, J.A. 1974. Blood lead values in pregnant women and their offspring. Am J Obstet and Gynecol 119:508–511.

Gillet, J.A. 1955. An outbreak of lead poisoning in the Canklow district of Rotterdam. Lancet 1:1118–1121.

Goyer, R.A. 1971. Lead and the kidney. Curr Top Pathol 55:147–176.

Goyer, R.A. and Wilson, M. 1975. Lead induced inclusion bodies, results of EDTA treatment. Lab Invest 32:149–156.

Haeger-Aronsen, B., Stathers, F. and Swahn, G. 1968. Hereditary coproporphyria: Study of a Swedish family. Ann Intern Med 69:221–227.

Lamola, A.A. and Yamane, T. 1974. Zinc protoporphyrin in the erythrocytes of patients with lead intoxication and iron deficiency anemia. Science 186:936–938.

Morris, H.P., Laug, E.P., Morris, H.J. and Grant, R.L. 1938. The growth and reproduction of rats fed diets containing lead acetate and arsenic trioxide and the lead and arsenic contents of newborn and suckling mice. J Pharmacol Exp Ther 64:420–445.

Muro, L.A. and Goyer, R.A. 1969. Chromosome damage in experimental lead poisoning. Arch Pathol 87:660–663.

Nishimura, H. 1964. In Chemistry and Prevention of Congenital Anomalies, page 13. Thomas, Springfield, Ill.

Oliver, T. 1914. Lead Poisoning. Lewis, London.

O'Riordan, M.L. and Evans, H.J. 1974. Absence of significant chromosome damage in males occupationally exposed to lead. Nature 247:50–53.

Piper, W.N. and Tephyl, T.R. 1974. Differential inhibition of erythrocyte and hepatic uroporphyrinogen 1 synthetase activity by lead. Life Sciences 14:873–876.

Potter, E.L. 1961. In Pathology of the Fetus and Newborn, Vol. 2, p. 168. Year Book Publ., Chicago, Ill.

Pueschel, S.M., Kopito, L. and Schwachman, H. 1972. A screening and follow-up study of children with an increased lead burden. J Am Med Assoc 222:462–466.

Schwanitz, G., Lehnert, G. and Gebhart, E. 1970. Chromosomenschaden bei beruflicher Bleibelastung. Deut Med Wochenschr 95:1636–1641.

Seppalainen, A.M., Tola, S., Hernberg, S. and Kock, B. 1975. Subclinical neuropathy at "safe" levels of lead exposure. Arch Environ Health 30:180–183.

Seto, D. and Freeman, J.M. 1964. Lead neuropathy in childhood. Amer J Dis Child 107:337–342.

Stowe, H.D. and Goyer, R.A. 1971. The reproductive ability and progeny of F, lead-toxic rats. Fert Steril 22:755–760.

Thomas, H.M. 1904. A case of generalized lead paralysis, with a review of the cases of lead palsy seen in the hospital. Johns Hopkins Hosp. Bull 15:209–212.

Vermande-Van Eck, G.J. and Meigs, J.W. 1960. Changes in the ovary of the Rhesus monkey after chronic lead intoxication. Fert Steril 11:223–234.

Wedeen, R.P., Maesaka, J.K., Weiner, B., Lipat, E.A., Lyons, M.M., Vitale, L.F. and Joselow, M.M. 1975. Occupational lead nephropathy. Am J Med 59:630–641.

Weller, C.V. 1951. The blastophtoric effect of chronic lead poisoning. J Med Res 33:271–293.

WHO 1977. Environ Health Criteria 3, Lead, Geneva.

Wilson, V.K., Thomson, M.L. and Dent, C.E. 1953. Aminoaciduria in lead poisoning. A case in childhood. Lancet 2:66–68.

4. Sub-encephalopathic Lead Poisoning: Central Nervous System Effects in Children

Evan Charney

Introduction

The purpose of this chapter is to assess the evidence that low level lead ingestion in children is harmful to central nervous system functioning. There has been remarkable progress over the past twenty years in eliminating frank lead encephalopathy. We see only a fraction of the number of children who used to present with unequivocal and serious central nervous system involvement from chronic lead ingestion. Bringing this serious hazard under control is indeed a tribute to the clinicians, biochemists, public health personnel and those in government who have helped define the disease, developed and instituted widespread screening techniques for its identification and implemented effective legal procedures to render homes safe for occupancy. Despite this success, we are left with a vexing issue: are the tens of thousands of overtly asymptomatic children we now identify with mildly elevated blood lead levels already suffering from a disease, or do they just represent a high risk group on whom preventive efforts can be focused to avert serious encephalopathy? If these children merit only careful monitoring, then the situation is in fact under good control; we have reduced the ''disease'' to a rarity. On the other hand, if these children are already damaged, then there is a serious epidemic in this country, one that may affect upwards of 100,000 children. Moreover, the disease selectively affects the children of the poor and the educationally disadvantaged, certainly those least able to cope with the impact of subtle brain damage. The distinction is an important one. Our present screening, treatment and environmental control program is effective in preventing major lead encephalopathy. It is woefully inadequate to prevent or treat subencephalopathic lead poisoning.

In considering this issue, we will briefly review the nature of the toxicity in severe lead encephalopathy, consider why the question of milder damage has been difficult to answer and then consider studies, particularly those conducted over the past decade, which have attempted to clarify the issue.

There seems to be little question that children who recover from frank lead encephalopathy have an increased risk for residual damage, characterized by varying degrees of mental retardation and less than expected intellectual performance (Perlstein and Attala, 1966; Mellins and Jenkins, 1955; Byers and Lord, 1943). Although these early studies were not controlled rigorously, the data appear consistent with the residual effects of encephalopathy due to infection, toxins and trauma. Moreover, it has been demonstrated (Goldstein et al., 1974) that lead begins to be taken up by the brain at very low blood levels and is retained in the brain as the blood level falls, similar to lead metabolism of other soft tissues. This lack of a threshold for brain lead would suggest that any associated brain damage might be on a continuum as well. Against this notion, however, is the evidence that severe lead encephalopathy is due in large part to brain edema caused by capillary damage and exudation, principally in the cerebellar area. It is unlikely that significant brain edema occurs at sub-encephalopathic levels. By this reasoning, a minimally increased body lead burden should not be assumed automatically to result in long term central nervous system (CNS) effects, at least by that mechanism alone.

In reviewing the studies on children, it is evident that it has been extremely difficult to determine clearly whether sub-encephalopathic lead intoxication results in long term sequelae. Despite a considerable range of studies over several decades, an unequivocal answer eludes us. Over and above the methodologic problems of any single study there are several other reasons for this dilemma:

1. *There Has Not Been a Single Accepted Indicator of Body Lead Exposure.* Whole blood lead, erythrocyte protoporphyrin, urinary excretion of lead following chelation and hair and tooth lead levels have been used, individually and in combination, to define the extent of the body lead burden. Blood lead and erythrocyte protoporphyrin reflect exposure at a given time and do not indicate the magnitude of exposure in years past. The technical problems of hair analysis to date have precluded its use beyond relatively crude estimates of exposure. Tooth dentine levels confirm exposure in the past but as yet do not define the exact time when the exposure occurred, nor have they been correlated prospectively with blood levels so that we may infer the level of exposure that is hazardous.

2. *There Is Not Agreement about Whether There Is a Particular Age, Duration or Intensity of Exposure during Childhood that Particularly Increases the Risk of Mild Encephalopathy.* There may be subgroups at real risk that are not identified among all those with evidence of past exposure to excess lead.

3. *The Outcome Measure—the Dependent Variable—Is Not Clearly Defined.* A variety of measures of "brain damage" have been employed, again without agreement as to the exact nature of that damage. Thus, measures of IQ, measures of general cognitive development and a host of behavioral measures with varying degrees of validation have been employed. Measures of neurologic and specific psychomotor function have also been used, including peripheral nerve conduction time, visual attention and memory, "soft" neurologic signs and the like. In all, perhaps 50 or more separate measures of the potential CNS effects have been employed in various studies and rarely has the same battery been used in more than one study.

4. *Confounding Variables Have Been Hard to Control For.* The population at risk for subtle brain damage from lead is the same population most likely to be exposed to poor home environment, nutritional deficiencies, low parental IQ and inadequate cognitive stimulation. All of these are known correlates of poor intellectual and behavioral performance in later childhood. It is virtually impossible in retrospective studies to determine whether lead exposure was a cause or a consequence of damage in such circumstances.

In short, with imprecise measures of the intensity and duration of the lead exposure, with varying definitions of the nature of the insult and with a host of confounding variables, it is perhaps not surprising that subtle brain effects have been difficult to define with precision.

With these caveats, let us turn to a review of the studies. One group of investigations has focused on the link between lead exposure, mental retardation and hyperactivity. Moncrieff et al. (1964) noted that blood lead concentrations were frequently elevated in mentally subnormal children. In 1968 Bicknell et al. showed that blood levels were elevated in retarded children with pica but were not elevated in retarded children without pica; he speculated that it was the pica that was responsible for lead ingestion in already mentally subnormal children. A series of studies by David et al. (1976) also has attempted to link retardation and blood lead levels. In a subgroup of mildly retarded children in whom an etiology other than lead poisoning was known or suspected, blood lead levels averaged 18.8 μg/dl compared to an average level of 25.5 μg/dl in comparable retarded children without an etiology. Although David concluded that a blood lead level of 25 μg/dl might therefore be hazardous, it would be more logical to assume that if a causal link existed it would be that significantly higher earlier lead levels in those children were responsible for the damage. However, a host of other potentially confounding factors (e.g., family background and IQ, adequacy of early histories, presence of pica) makes it difficult to draw any strong conclusions from these studies.

Several studies from Glasgow, Scotland, are more intriguing (Moore et al., 1977; Beattie et al., 1975). From an analysis of dried blood on phenylketonuria (PKU) cards obtained in the neonatal period, it was determined that blood lead values were slightly but significantly higher in retarded children as compared to controls. The investigators also noted a somewhat higher average lead content in the drinking water in homes where mothers of the retarded children had lived during pregnancy and during the child's first year of life than in the drinking water of control families. Although the study did identify true differences in mean blood and drinking water values, these differences were slight, with a great deal of overlap in the two groups studied. It is difficult to attribute the major retardation in these cases to the rather minor differences in lead exposure.

David et al. (1972, 1976, 1977) have also published a series of articles linking hyperactivity in childhood to lead ingestion. They initially demonstrated a minimally elevated blood lead in hyperactive children where no cause could be ascertained compared to hyperactive children with some identified cause (mean values 26 versus 23 μg/dl). In a subsequent small scale study, hyperactive children with no known cause for their hyperactivity were given chelation therapy for four weeks. These children showed an improvement in behavior by a teacher rating scale, compared to chelated children with some cause for their hyperactivity, which was therefore not presumably attributable to lead. Methodologic problems were serious in this study, including use of incompletely standardized behavioral measures, rather minor differences in scores between groups on those scales and a question of whether observers were blind to the children's blood lead values. At most these data suggest some association between lead ingestion and hyperactivity, but a causal link is harder to accept. It is at least equally likely that hyperactive children acquire more lead from their environment through pica and hand contamination with lead dust than do nonhyperactive children and that the elevated lead values are a result rather than a cause of the hyperactivity.

There have been a series of studies conducted on children exposed to lead from fallout of particulate matter from a lead smelter (Lansdowne et al., 1974; Landrigan et al., 1975; McNeil and Ptasnik, 1975; Hebel et al., 1976). Ingestion in these cases is presumably due to a combination of direct inhalation, contamination of interior dust and outside soil and subsequent direct ingestion by mouthing lead dust on contaminated hands or toys and household objects. Theoretically, these studies should have a substantial advantage over other retrospective studies in that the population of children was not selected for a deteriorated home environment and concomitant social and family disorganization, factors which themselves may cause behavioral and intellectual impairment. This advantage would be most valid if the lead burden was due entirely to inhalation of lead dust (presumably affecting all households regardless of social status) and less true if ingestion was by mouthing of contaminated dust in dirtier homes and chronic pica for soil. Unfortunately, the studies do not tease out these variables.

The most carefully studied subjects were drawn from the El Paso-Smeltertown area, where a lead-emitting smelter contaminated the area for a number of years. Landrigan and associates (1975) studied 46 children 3 to 15 yr of age with elevated blood lead levels, most exposed since birth, and compared them to 78 control children well matched for age, socioeconomic status (SES), ethnicity and proximity to the smelter. A variety of psychological and neurologic tests were done blindly. In the lead-exposed group, the performance portion of the IQ test (Wechsler Intelligence Scale for Children or Wechsler Preschool and Primary Scale for Intelligence) was significantly less (95 versus 103) and finger tapping rate was slower. Both differences persisted even when the data were controlled for pica in the child. A second study of a largely different group of children from the El Paso-Smeltertown area performed shortly after they moved out of Smeltertown but using controls from a different area showed absolutely no differences between lead-exposed and control subjects on similar (but not identical) variables (McNeil and Ptasnik, 1975). A review of these two studies (and a third) of the Smeltertown data by Muir (1978) found them inconclusive. There are some methodologic problems in both studies and a question in the Landrigan data of just why control subjects should have had such a relatively high performance IQ for a deprived population. Unfortunately, additional smelter studies from Birmingham, Manchester and London in England and from Idaho are all similarly inconclusive, with perhaps a slight tendency for lead-exposed subjects to demonstrate minimally lower IQ scores. It is possible that impairment in some children could have preceded and perhaps predisposed to lead ingestion, particularly by the oral route. Where differences were evident it may be that other toxins contained in the smelter fallout were responsible. Certainly, the differences that were evident in these studies were hardly dramatic ones.

De La Burde and Choate (1972, 1975), from the Medical College of Virginia, followed 67 1- to 3-yr-olds with blood levels of 40 to 100 μg/dl through ages 7 to 8 and compared them to 70 control children without pica from recently built homes in good repair. The controls were well matched for age, SES and maternal IQ. Although no lead levels were available initially on control subjects, tooth lead levels on a number of control patients were significantly lower than on study subjects. The children were tested at 4 years of age and again at 7 to 8 years using a variety of psychological, neurological and school evaluations all done blindly by observers. Slight IQ differences favored the controls (94 versus 89), but more impressive was the increase in school failure and behavioral problems in the lead-exposed group (25 to 28% so affected compared to 4 to 6% of controls). These data are suggestive, but it is still hard to identify lead as the sole responsible factor since those from better homes may differ in ways other than parental IQ and SES, which may lead in turn to better school performance.

Several other studies (Baloh et al., 1975; Kotok, 1977; Sachs et al., 1978) have failed to show differences between experimental and control children, using different measures of behavioral and psychological functioning.

The most impressive study to date suggesting significant impairment of lead-exposed children was conducted by Needleman (1979). Deciduous teeth were collected from 3300 first and second grade students in Chelsea and Somerville, Massachusetts. The 58 children with the highest and 100 children with the lowest dentine lead levels were compared on an extensive battery of psychological tests and teacher performance ratings. Teacher ratings were also available on 2146 children in whom dentine lead levels were known. Children with high tooth levels scored lower on the verbal portion of WISC and lower on most items of the teacher rating scale than did controls. Most astonishing was the close correlation between teacher ratings and lead levels with the "frequency of negative teacher ratings increasing with increasing dentine lead levels . . . not limited to the group with the highest level." Although the study does not rule out the possibility that antecedent impairment leads both to lead ingestion and poor school performance (the classic confounder of all of these studies), it is striking that increments of tooth lead burden are closely correlated with decrements in school performance, a finding that if true would strongly implicate Pb as a causal factor.

Summary

What conclusions can be reached about the hazard of sub-encephalopathic lead ingestion? Certainly, no single study has been ideal in that it has been prospective, has documented a group of children to be similar in all of the principal confounding variables at birth and then has observed the effect of lead ingestion as it occurs. For ethical reasons such a study is impossible to conduct. The data certainly do not provide assurance that low-level lead absorbtion is not hazardous. The proof of absence of a hazard is difficult, indeed. The data available to date do suggest that there is reason for concern; blood lead levels of 40 to 60 µg/dl during early childhood appear to be associated with a 2- to 6-point reduction in IQ scores and with a less easy to document but suggestive negative effect on school performance. An excellent recent review by Rutter (1980) reaches a similar conclusion. Needleman's work (1979) in particular merits replication, since it represents a well designed study with clear detrimental effects on the exposed children.

However, the present information still leaves major gaps in our understanding of the problem. It is most important to determine at what age and at what levels of body lead burden the hazard becomes manifest. If there is a minimal but definite handicap associated with low-level ingestion among a large group of exposed children, it is quite possible that a particular subset of those children are especially affected, perhaps selected by intensity or duration of exposure at key points in development.

At a minimum these data suggest that we must continue to be vigorous in identifying families at risk and in separating children from their source of lead promptly. To extend significantly the scope and nature of present lead poisoning efforts does not appear warranted by the data now available. To do less than what is done at present, to curtail or to relax our current programs would be equally imprudent.

References

Baloh, R., Sturm, R., Green, B. and Gelser, G. 1975. Neuropsychological effects of chronic asymptomatic increased lead absorption. Arch Neurol 32:326–330.

Beattie, A.D., Moore, M.R., Goldberg, A., Finlayson, M.J.W., Graham, J.F., Mackie, E.M., Main, J.D., McLaren, D.A., Murdoch, R.M. and Steward, G.T. 1975. Role of chronic low-level lead exposure in the aetiology of mental retardation. Lancet 1:589–592.

Bicknell, D.J., Clayton, B.E. and Delves, H.T. 1968. Lead in mentally retarded children. J Ment Defic Res 12:282.

Byers, R.K. and Lord, E.E. 1943. Late effects of lead poisoning on mental development. Amer J Dis Child 66:471–494.

David, O.J., Clark, J. and Voeller, K. 1972. Lead and hyperactivity. Lancet 2:900–903.

David, O.J., Hoffman, S., McGann, B., Sverd, J. and Clark, J. 1976. Low lead levels and mental retardation. Lancet 2:1376–1379.

David, O.J., Sverd, J. and Clark, J. 1977. Lead and hyperactivity: lead levels among hyperactive children. J Abnorm Child Psych 5:405–416.

De La Burde, B. and Choate, M.S. 1972. Does asymptomatic lead exposure in children have latent sequelae? J Pediatr 81:1088-1091.

De La Burde, B. and Choate, M.S. 1975. Early asymptomatic lead exposure and development at school age. J. Pediatr 87:638–642.

Goldstein, G.W., Asbury, A. and Diamond, I. 1974. Pathogenesis of lead encephalopathy. Arch Neurol 31:382–389.

Hebel, J.R., Kinch, D. and Armstrong, E. 1976. Mental capability of children exposed to lead pollution. Brit J Prev Soc Med 30:170–174

Kotok, D. 1977. Development of children with elevated blood lead levels: A controlled study. J Pediatr 80:57–61.

Landrigan, P.G., Gehlback, S.H., Rosenblum, B.F., Shoults, J.M., Candelaria, R.M., Barthel, W.R., Liddle, J.A., Smrek, A., Staehling, M.W. and Sanders, J.F. 1975. Epidemic lead absorption near an ore smelter: The role of particulate lead. New Engl J Med 282:123–129.

Lansdowne, R.G., Shepherd, J., Clayton, B.E., Delves, H.T., Graham, P.J. and Turner, W.C. 1974. Blood lead levels, behaviour and intelligence: A population study. Lancet 1:538–541.

McNeil, J.L. and Ptasnik, J.S. 1975. Draft, Final Report, Project LH-208: Epidemiological Study of a Lead Contaminated Area. International Lead and Zinc Research Organization.

Mellins, R.B. and Jenkins, C.D. 1955. Epidemiological and psychological study of lead poisoning in children. JAMA 158:15–20.

Moncrieff, A.A., Koumides, O.P., Clayton, B.E., Patrick, A.D., Renwick, A.G.C. and Roberts, G.C. 1964. Lead poisoning in children. Arch Dis Child 39:1–13.

Moore, M.R., Meredith, P.A. and Goldberg, A. 1977. A retrospective analysis of blood lead in mentally retarded children. Lancet 1:717–719.

Muir, W. 1978. Proceedings of the International Conference on Heavy Metals in the Environment. Toronto. U.S. Government Printing Office, 757–140/6681.

Needleman, H.L., Grunnoe C.E., Leviton, A., Reed, R., Peresie, H., Maher, C. and Barretti, P.1979. Deficits in psychological and classroom performance of children with elevated dentive levels. New Engl J Med 300:689-695.

Perlstein, M.A. and Attala, R. 1966. Neurologic sequelae of plumbism in children. Clin Pediatr 5:292–298.

Ratcliffe, J.M. 1977. Developmental and behavioural functions in young children with elevated blood lead levels. Brit J Prev Soc Med 31:258–264.

Rutter, M. 1980. Raised lead levels and impaired cognitive/behavioural functioning: A review of the evidence. Devel Med Child Neurol (suppl.) 22:1–23.

Sachs, H.K., Drall, V., McCaughran, D.A., Rozenfeld, I.H., Youngsmith, N., Growe, G., Lazar, B., Novar, L., O'Connel, L. and Rayson, B. 1978. IQ following treatment of lead poisoning: A patient-sibling comparison. J Pediatr 93:428–431.

Wegner, G. (Ed.) 1976. Shoshone Lead Health Project. Idaho Department of Health and Welfare. Boise.

5. Developmental Neurotoxicity of Lead: Experimental Studies

Lawrence W. Reiter

Introduction

It is generally accepted that children represent the population at high risk to lead exposure. However, prior to 1965, the animal literature on lead-induced cerebral dysfunction was limited. This limitation stemmed from the lack of an appropriate animal model which exhibited unequivocal neurological changes comparable to the human clinical cases of lead encephalopathy. A breakthrough in the development of an experimental model exhibiting central nervous system (CNS) morphological alterations similar to those in children with lead encephalopathy occurred when Pentschew (1965) and Pentschew and Garro (1966) showed that morphological changes in the CNS of neonatal rats were produced when lead was transmitted to the suckling pup via the maternal milk. Ninety per cent of the pups developed paraplegia between 23 and 29 days of age; 85 to 90% of the paraplegic animals died during this period. Neuropathological examination revealed capillary activation, glial proliferation and hemorrhages primarily in the cerebellum and striatum. The authors concluded that lead encephalopathy in the suckling rat was caused by a disorder in the permeability of capillaries, a dysoric encephalopathy. Further verification of the dysoric nature of lead encephalopathy in the suckling rat was provided by Lambert et al. (1967), who administered either Thorotrast or trypan blue. Neither of these compounds normally penetrates the blood-brain barrier; however, in lead-poisoned rats both compounds were found in the cerebellum, striatum, occipital lobes and spinal cord.

Since the initial description of lead encephalopathy in the rat, several investigators have replicated this finding, including Thomas et al. (1971), Michaelson and Sauerhoff (1974) and Krigman and Hogan (1974).

Lead encephalopathy in the mouse was first described by Rosenblum and Johnson (1968), who also used the suckling animal. In contrast to the rat brain, the striatum and cerebellum of the mice fed either 0.5 or 1% lead carbonate displayed only faint staining with trypan blue (except for a darkly stained cerebellum in a single animal). In addition, paralysis was a rare finding. These authors concluded that no cerebral edema or focal destructive lesions were found in the mouse brain and, therefore, the histological response of the suckling mouse exposed to lead differed from that seen in the suckling rat. These differences in the neuropathological response to lead are probably not attributable to different exposure levels (4% lead carbonate in the rat versus 1% in the mouse), since the food consumption per unit body weight was three to four times greater in the mouse than in the rat. Therefore, at high exposure levels, the histological changes associated with lead encephalopathy vary among species and are characterized by their relative involvement of neuronal degeneration and vasculopathy.

Since the initial description of lead encephalopathy in the rat, considerable research has focused on more closely defining the neurotoxicity of lead at sub-encephalopathic exposure levels. A comprehensive review of the literature on the neurobehavioral effects of developmental lead exposure is beyond the scope of this paper; extensive reviews are available elsewhere (Damstra, 1977; WHO, 1977; EPA, 1977; Bornschein et al., 1980). Instead, this paper will consider some general biochemical properties of lead which may contribute to its neurotoxicity, and results which demonstrate that perinatal lead exposure disrupts nervous system development. First, some general aspects of nervous system development will be considered.

CNS Development

In most mammalian species, the development of the nervous system occurs over a protracted period of time. In general, this process begins early in gestation, during the period of organogenesis, and extends into the postnatal period. The three basic processes of CNS development are cell division, migration and differentiation. The nervous system, however, is not a simple, homogeneous structure. Consequently, different neural structures undergo development at different times and at differential rates. To a great extent, birth may be thought of as a random event relative to the development of the mammalian nervous system. Dobbing (1970a), using deoxyribonucleic acid (DNA) as a measure of cellularity, calculated the rates of CNS development in various species relative to parturition. The period of rapid cell division, which he termed the ''brain growth-spurt," varied from species to species. The nervous system of the guinea pig, for example, develops prenatally whereas the rapid growth-spurt of the rat occurs postnatally. However, the overall rate of cell division can be misleading since it represents both neuronal and glial growth and does not reflect the heterogeneity of the CNS nor the differential periods during which different cells divide. For example, neurons multiply early in development so that adult levels are achieved largely before these growth-spurts begin. Neuronal division is essentially complete by 42 days of gestation in the guinea pig, by the second day postnatally in the rat and by 25 weeks of gestation in man (Dobbing, 1970b). However, since the greatest number of brain cells are glia, the growth-spurts reported by Dobbing are more indicative of the mitotic activity in these support cells, which occurs concurrently with the differentiation of axonal and dendritic processes of neurons.

Dobbing (1970b) has formulated a "critical period" hypothesis to describe the vulnerability of the developing brain to undernutrition. This hypothesis states that the brain is likely to be most vulnerable to undernutrition during the period of the brain growth-spurt. Two corollaries to this hypothesis are that the required severity of the undernutrition decreases as one approaches the period of rapid growth and that undernutrition at any stage of development will produce differential effects because of the differential rates of growth in various brain regions.

Although the critical periods hypothesis was formulated to explain the neurobehavioral consequences of undernutrition during CNS development, it may also apply to many of the neurotoxic effects seen following perinatal exposure to chemicals. The hypothesis to be developed here is that the developmental neurotoxicity of lead results from the disruption of normal developmental processes. Several biochemical processes which are vital to normal cell function are disrupted by lead and it is postulated that these effects account for the neurobehavioral consequences of lead exposure. Since these biochemical effects are nonspecific, they will affect all cells in the brain. Therefore, the functional consequences of this early insult will depend on both the period and the level of lead exposure.

Table 1.   Inhibition of brain mitochondrial respiration.

A   Bull et al. (1975)
     Inhibition of K^+-stimulated respiration
     in rat cerebral cortex slices

B   Brierley (1977)
     Mitochondria bind lead
     Inhibits succinate oxidation

C   Holtzman et al. (1978)
     Inhibition of ADP-dependent respiration
     Inhibition of NAD-linked dehydrogenases
     Adult and immature rat brain mitochondria are equally sensitive

Biochemical Effects of Lead

Three biochemical effects of lead will be discussed: inhibition of mitochondrial respiration; nonspecific enzyme inhibition and competitive inhibition of calcium.

Inhibition of Mitochondrial Respiration

Lead exposure both in vivo and in vitro has been shown to inhibit brain mitochondrial respiration (Table 1). Bull et al. (1975) reported inhibition of potassium-stimulated respiration in rat cerebral cortical slices following subacute administration of lead. This inhibition was produced by an external exposure which resulted in a mean blood lead level of 72 μg/dl and a mean brain level of 41 ppm. A similar inhibition was observed when mitochondria were exposed in vitro to 67 μM of lead.

Brierley (1977) found that lead bound in a quantitative fashion to mitochondria isolated from either heart or brain and that exposure of isolated mitochondria to lead resulted in inhibition of succinate oxidation. Holtzman et al. (1978) reported that lead inhibited respiration dependent upon adenosine diphosphate (ADP) as well as dehydrogenases linked to nicotinamide adenosine diphosphate (NAD). Mitochondria isolated from adult and immature rat brains were equally sensitive to lead.

Table 2.   Enzymes affected by lead in animal studies.

Reference	Enzyme	Effect
Ulmer and Vallee (1969)	Lipoamide dehydrogenase	Inhibited
Muro and Goyer (1969)	DNAase	Enhanced
Minden et al. (1964)	Serum glutamic oxaloacetic transaminase (SGOT)	Enhanced and transitory
	Serum glutamic pyruvic transaminase (SGPT)	Enhanced and transitory
	Serum alkaline phosphatase (AP)	Lowered
	Erythrocyte and liver AP	Variable
	Acid phosphatase	Quenched or markedly inhibited
Soldatovic and Petrovic (1963)	Catalase	Variable
Geleriu and Straus (1972)	Cholinesterase	Markedly inhibited
Apostolov et al. (1976)	α-Mannosidase	Increased
	β-Acetyl glucosaminadase	Increased
Innaccone et al. (1974)	Succinate oxidase	Decreased
	Cytochrome c reductase	Decreased
	Glutamate dehydrogenase	Decreased
	Cytochrome oxidase	Decreased
Nathanson and Bloom (1975)	Adenyl cyclase	Decreased
Yamamoto et al. (1975)	β-Glucuronidase	Elevated
	β-Galactosidase	Elevated

Several investigators have demonstrated, therefore, that lead exposure both in vivo and in vitro inhibits mitochondrial respiration. This disruption of energy metabolism would be expected to produce dramatic effects on the developing, metabolically active nervous system.

Enzyme Inhibition

A variety of enzymes are known to be sensitive to lead exposure. Table 2 lists a number of enzymes affected by lead exposure in animals. A more extensive description of these effects is found elsewhere (EPA, 1977). The point here is that lead interferes with the normal activity of a wide variety of enzyme systems. As with several other metals, lead has a high affinity for various complexing groups such as the imidazole nitrogen, cysteine sulfhydryl and the e-amino·group of lysine. An effect may be imparted, therefore, by perturbation of the structural integrity of enzymes or by the disruption of substrate-enzyme binding.

Inhibition of Calcium

Lead has also been shown in a variety of biological systems to inhibit calcium competitively (Table 3). Since calcium is required for normal neurotransmitter release, this competition would be expected to interfere with synaptic transmission. Kostial and Vouk (1957) first demonstrated this effect using the cat superior cervical ganglion. They found that the postsynaptic response to presynaptic stimulation was reduced when lead was added to the bathing solution and that this inhibition was reversed by excess calcium. Kober and Cooper (1976), using the frog sympathetic ganglion, demonstrated that the spike-evoked entry of calcium into the presynaptic terminals was blocked by lead and that this effect

Table 3.   Competitive inhibition of calcium.

A   Synaptic transmission

 1. Kostial and Vouk (1957). Lead blocks in vitro transmission in cat superior cervical ganglion. Reversed by excess calcium.
 2. Kober and Cooper (1976). Lead blocks spike evoked entry of calcium into presynaptic terminals in frog sympathetic ganglion.
 3. Cooper and Steinberg (1977). Lead blocks neural transmission in adrenergic synapses in rabbit saphenous artery. Reversed by excess calcium.
 4. Carroll et al. (1977). Lead blocks K-stimulated release of acetylcholine in cortical minces from mice chronically exposed to lead.

B   Choline uptake

Silbergeld (1977). Lead inhibits high affinity choline uptake. Effect mimicked by reduced calcium.

was reversed by calcium. Their kinetic data demonstrated that this effect was due to competitive inhibition.

Adrenergic synapses are also affected by lead as was shown by Cooper and Steinberg (1977) using the rabbit saphenous artery. As with the cholinergic synapse, this effect was reversed by calcium. Finally, Carroll and co-workers (1977) demonstrated that mice chronically exposed to lead in vivo showed a reduction in potassium-stimulated release of both choline and acetylcholine from cortical minces.

A second calcium-dependent system, the high affinity choline uptake system, was shown by Silbergeld (1977) to be inhibited by lead exposure in vitro. This effect was mimicked by reducing the calcium concentration in the incubation medium.

To summarize, data obtained from a variety of mammalian and nonmammalian neural tissues demonstrate that lead competitively inhibits the effects of calcium both in vivo and in vitro. The extent to which this competition interferes with normal neuronal development remains to be determined.

Developmental Neurotoxicity of Lead

Numerous investigators have examined the effects of perinatal lead exposure on development in the rodent using a variety of neurological, physiological and biochemical endpoints. Table 4 lists a number of representative developmental parameters which have been evaluated. The table is limited to experiments which employed external exposures producing blood lead levels below 100 μg/dl. In addition, either lead exposure in these experiments was not associated with undernutrition of the offspring or adequate controls for the reduced growth were provided.

In all studies listed in Table 4, lead exposure produced a delay in normal maturation. Delays were observed in the development of the righting reflex, sexual maturation in females (as indicated by the age at vaginal opening), thermoregulation, the visual evoked potential, cerebral cytochrome concentrations and cerebral synaptogenesis.

Table 4. Developmental delays associated with lead exposure in the rodent.

1. Righting reflex. Reiter et al. (1975); Kimmel et al. (1976).
2. Sexual maturation (females). Kimmel et al. (1976); Gray and Reiter (1977).
3. Thermoregulation. Fox (1979).
4. Visual evoked potential. Fox et al. (1977).
5. Cerebral cytochrome concentrations. Bull et al. (1979).
6. Cerebral synaptogenesis. McCauley et al. (1979).

Table 5. The effect of lead and/or undernutrition on age at development of righting reflex in the rat. Regression analysis indicated a significant effect of lead ($p < .02$) and litter size ($p < .004$) (Reiter, unpublished data).

Litter Size	Dose of Lead		
	0	100 ppm	200 ppm
8	18.6 ± 0.1 ‡ (6)*	19.0 ± 0.4 (4)	19.4 ± 0.3 (4)
11	18.9 ± 0.2 (5)	19.4 ± 0.1 (5)	
14	19.4 ± 0.3 (5)		20.1 ± 0.2 (5)

*Number of litters tested (3 males and 3 females/litter).
‡ Age in days.

Table 5 illustrates the effects of perinatal lead exposure on development of the righting reflex in rats. On gestational day 2, lead exposure was initiated with levels of 0, 100 and 200 ppm in the drinking water. At 29 days of age, the offspring had blood lead levels of approximately 25 µg/dl. Litter size was used as an independent variable to evaluate the effects of early undernutrition on development. At parturition, litter size was adjusted to either 8, 11 or 14 pups. Pups reared in litters of 14 showed approximately a 25% reduction in growth during the period of lactation. Two combinations of litter size and lead exposure were also included in the experimental design. Both treatments caused a significant delay in the development of the righting reflex. In addition, the combination of high lead exposure and large litter size resulted in an additive delay in the development of this response. These results illustrate that undernutrition and early lead exposure produce additive effects resulting in a significant delay in neurological maturation.

Figure 1 is taken from Fox (1979) and illustrates the effects of neonatal lead exposure on the development of thermoregulation in the rat. Dams were exposed to 0.2% lead acetate in the drinking water beginning at parturition. This exposure produced blood lead levels of 89 µg/dl at 21 days of age and resulted in a significant delay in the development of thermoregulation measured as surface body temperature following 1 hr of isolation from the dam.

The third example of a lead-induced maturational delay is taken from McCauley et al. (1979) who evaluated synaptogensis in developing rat pups. Females were given 200 ppm lead in the drinking water from 14 days prior to breeding until weaning of the pups at 21 days of age, while controls received tap water. This exposure level produced blood lead levels of 36 µg/dl at 21 days of age.

Synaptogensis was measured using an ethanol-phosphotungstic acid stain which has been used previously to determine the density and maturity of cerebral synapses (Bloom, 1977). Synaptic structures were observed as an electron-dense band associated with varying numbers of electron-dense spots. The electron-dense band is associated with the postsynaptic membrane, whereas the electron-dense spots are presynaptic and are referred to as presynaptic dense projections (PDP). The average number of PDP has been shown to increase with the age of the animal (Bloom, 1977). Consequently, the average number of PDP may be used as an index of synaptic maturity. Figure 2 shows data from 15-day-old control and lead-exposed rat pups. Data are presented as the mean number of synaptic structures for synapses of varying complexity ranging from 0 to 6. Lead-exposed pups had fewer synaptic figures than control animals. This depression in synaptic figures was due primarily to fewer structures with PDP since there was little difference in the number of figures not associated with this structure (i.e., those with a synaptic complexity of zero). Structures with one, two and three presynaptic projections accounted for the bulk of differences in the total counts.

Summary and Conclusions

The present discussion has focused on experiments which demonstrate that perinatal lead exposure delays normal brain maturation. This maturational delay has been demonstrated using neurological, physiological, biochemical and morphological measurements and is associated with blood lead levels ranging from 25 to 89 μg/dl. No clear relationship between the period of exposure and effect has been established, since animals were exposed to lead either during gestation and lactation or during lactation alone. The results of Fox (1979) are of particular interest with regard to exposure level because his data indicate that within 2 days after initiating lead exposure, suckling pups showed a significant impairment of thermoregulation. Replication of these results should include measurements of lead during early life of the offspring to determine the lead levels associated with this effect.

Experimental results have tended to be more variable with studies that evaluate the effects of lead exposure on complex behavioral responses. Since complex behaviors are influenced by a variety of organismic and environmental factors, and since the neurotoxicity of lead likely results from nonspecific biochemical effects during development, the reports of conflicting behavioral effects of lead may reflect differences in experimental design, methods of lead exposure (both dose and period of exposure) and methods used to evaluate behavior. For example, in the 19 experiments reviewed in EPA's Lead Criteria Document (1977) which dealt with the effects of lead on motor activity, 10 different measures of activity were utilized. It is well known that methodology has a considerable influence on motor activity (Reiter and MacPhail, 1979) and therefore it is not surprising that considerable variability exists in the literature concerning the effects of lead on this behavioral endpoint.

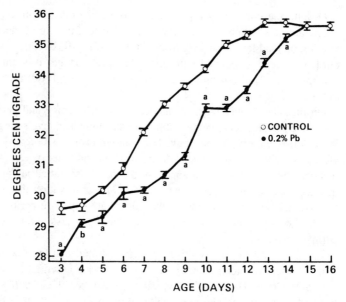

Fig. 1. Final body temperature of control and neonatally Pb-exposed rats following 69 min of isolation from dam. Points indicate means ± SE for 18 to 24 male rats. Initial temperature was the same for both groups, 35.7 ± 0.3°C. Ambient temperature was 22.0 ± 1.0°C. (Fox, 1979). Reprinted with permission of *Neurobehavioral Toxicology* 1 (Suppl.): 193-206.

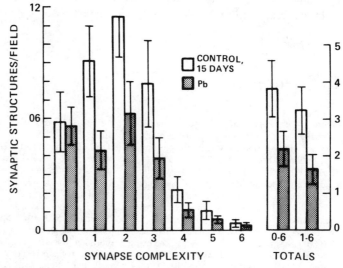

Fig. 2. Pb-induced suppression of synaptic figures in the 15-day-old rat cerebral cortex. Level of complexity was judged by the number of presynaptic dense projections. Results of seven control and seven Pb liters ± S.E.M. (McCauley et al., 1979). Reprinted with permission of *Neuropharmacology* 18:91-101.

Despite the conflicting reports on lead-induced changes in motor activity in young animals, when changes have been reported, they are generally associated with blood lead levels ranging from 170 to 550 μg/dl. Because of the high body burdens of lead associated with this behavioral change, it is unlikely to reflect asymptomatic lead poisoning (See Bornschein et al. (1980) for more extensive discussion).

On the other hand, experiments dealing with learning and performance have shown behavioral decrements at much lower blood lead levels ranging from 30 to 80 μg/dl. A variety of tasks have been shown to be disrupted by lead including electric shock avoidance, visual discrimination and other types of operant performance. These effects do not appear to be species-specific, having been reported in mice, rats, dogs, sheep and monkeys. The observation that these effects of lead on behavior persist beyond the immediate exposure period would suggest that lead produces permanent alterations in nervous system function as a result of perinatal exposure.

In summary, several studies have demonstrated that lead exposure interferes with a variety of biochemical processes which are essential for normal nervous system function. The neurobehavioral consequences of lead exposure, particularly the developmental consequences, may reflect a disruption of these biochemical processes (i.e., mitochondrial respiration, enzyme activity and calcium-dependent neurotransmitter release). Since these processes are common to all cells in the nervous system, the consequences of exposure may depend largely on the particular and perhaps unique conditions of a given experiment. Clearly, additional research is needed to evaluate this hypothesis.

References

Apostolov, I., Zapryanov, Z., and Gylybova, V. 1976. Activity of serum lysomal enzymes in rats with experimental lead poisoning. Bull Ex Biol Med Engl. Trans. 82:1337–1339.

Bloom, F.E. 1977. The formation of synaptic junctions in developing rat brain. In Structure and Function of Synapses. Pappas, G.D. and Purpura, D.P., Eds. pp. 101–119. Raven Press, New York.

Bornschein, R., Pearson, D. and Reiter, L. 1980. Behavioral effects of moderate lead exposure in children and animal models: Part 1, clinical studies; Part 2, animal studies. CRC Critical Reviews in Toxicology. 8:43–152.

Brierley, G.P. 1977. Effects of heavy metals on isolated mitochondria. In Biochemical Effects of Environmental Pollutant. Lee, S.D., Ed.

pp. 397–411. Ann Arbor Sci Publ Inc., Ann Arbor.

Bull, R., Lutkenhoff, S.D., McCarty, G.E. and Muller, R.G. 1979. Delays in the postnatal increase of cerebral cytochrome concentrations in lead-exposed rats. Neuropharmacol 18:83–92.

Bull, R.J., Stanaszek, P.M., O'Neill, J.S. and Lutkenhoff, S.D. 1975. Specificity of the effects of lead on brain energy metabolism for substrates donating a cytoplasmic reducing equivalent. Envir Health Persp 12:89–95.

Carroll, P.T., Silbergeld, E.K. and Goldberg, A.M. 1977. Alternations of central cholinergic functions by lead exposure. Biochem Pharmacol 28:397–402.

Cooper, G.P. and Steinberg, D. 1977. Effects of cadmium and lead on adrenergic neuromuscular transmission in the rabbit. Am J Physiol 232:C128–C131.

Damstra, T. 1977. Toxicological properties of lead. Environ Health Perspectives. 19:297–307.

Dobbing, J. 1970a. Undernutrition and the developing brain. In Developmental Neurobiology, Himwich, W.A., Ed. pp 241–261 Charles C Thomas, Springfield.

Dobbing, J. 1970b. Undernutrition and the developing brain: The relevance of animal models to the human problem. Amer J Dis Child. 120:411–415.

EPA Air Quality Criteria for Lead. 1977. U.S. Environmental Protection Agency. U.S. Government Printing Office. No. EPA-600/8-77-017.

Fox, D.A. 1979. Physiological and neurobehavioral alterations during development in lead exposed rats. Neurobehav Toxicol 1(Suppl 1):193–206.

Fox, D., Lewkowski, J. and Cooper, G. 1977. Acute and chronic effects of neonatal lead exposure on development of the visual evoked response in rats. Toxic Appl Pharmacol 40:449–461.

Geleriu, R. and Straus, H. 1972. Effects of lead administered with goitrogenic agents (thiocyanates). In International Symposium, Environmental Health Aspects of Lead, pp. 249–254.

Gray, L.E. and Reiter, L.W. 1977. Lead-induced developmental and behavioral changes in the mouse. In 16th Annual Meeting of the Society of Toxicology, Toronto.

Holtzman, J., Hsu, S. and Mortell, P. 1978. In vitro effects of inorganic lead on isolated rat brain mitochondrial respiration. Neurochem Res 3:195–206.

Innaccone, A., Boscolo, P., Bertoli, E. and Bombardieri, G. 1974. In vitro effects of lead on enzymatic activities of rabbit kidney mitochondria. Experientia 30:467–468.

Kimmel, C.A., Grant, L.D. and Sloan, C.S. 1976. Chronic lead exposure: Assessment of developmental toxicity. Teratol 13:27A.

Kober, T.E. and Cooper, G.P. 1976. Lead competitively inhibits calcium dependent synaptic transmission in the bullfrog sympathetic ganglion. Nature 262:704–705.

Kostial, K. and Vouk, V.B. 1957. Lead ions and synaptic transmission in the superior cervical ganglion of the cat. Brit J Pharm 12:219–222.

Krigman, M.R. and Hogan, E.L. 1974. Effect of lead intoxication on the postnatal growth of the rat nervous system. Envir Health Persp 7:187–199.

Lambert, P., Garro, F. and Pentschew, A. 1967. Lead encephalopathy in the suckling rat. In Proc Symp on Edema, Vienna. 207–222.

McCauley, P.T., Bull, R.J. and Lutkenhoff, S.D. 1979. Association of alterations in energy metabolism with lead-induced delays in rat cerebral cortical development. Neuropharmacol 18:91–101.

Michaelson, I.A. and Sauerhoff, M.W. 1974. An improved model of lead-induced brain dysfunction in the suckling rat. Toxicol Appl Pharmacol 28:88–96.

Minden, H., Zegarski, W. and Rothe, P. 1964. Fermentuntersuchungen bei experimenteller bleivergiftung. Int Arch Gewerbepathol Gewerbehyg 20:461–470. Cited in Waldron, H.A. and Stofen, D. 1974. Sub-clinical Lead Poisoning. Academic Press, New York.

Muro, L.A. and Goyer, R.A. 1969. Chromosome damage in experimental lead poisoning. Arch Pathol 87:660–663.

Nathanson, J.A. and Bloom, F.E. 1975. Lead-induced inhibition of brain adenyl cyclase. Nature 255:419–420.

Pentschew, A. 1965. Morphology and morphogenesis of lead encephalopathy. Acta Neuropathol 5:133–160.

Pentschew, A. and Garro, F. 1966. Lead encephalo-myelopathy of the suckling rat and its implications on the porphyrinopathic nervous disease. Acta Neuropathol 6:266–278.

Reiter, L.W., Anderson, G.E., Laskey, J.W. and Cahill, D.F. 1975. Developmental and behavioral changes in the rat during chronic exposure to lead. Environ Health Perspec 12:119–123.

Reiter, L.W. and MacPhail, R.C. 1979. Motor activity: A survey of methods with potential use in toxicity testing. Neurobehavioral Toxicol 1(Suppl 1):53–66.

Rosenblum, W.I. and Johnson, M.G. 1968. Neuropathologic changes produced in suckling mice by adding lead to the maternal diet. Arch Path 85:640–648.

Silbergeld, E.K. 1977. Interactions of lead and calcium on the synaptosomal uptake of dopamine and choline. Life Sci 20:309–318.

Soldatovic, D. and Petrovic, D. 1963. Influence of lead on enzyme activity in animals poisoned by small amounts of lead. Arch Farm 13:253–258.

Thomas, J.A., Dallenbach, F.D. and Thomas, M. 1971. Considerations of the development of experimental lead encephalopathy. Virch Arch Alot A Path Anat 352:61–74.

Ulmer, D.D. and Vallee, B.L. 1969. Effects of lead on biochemical systems. In Trace Substances in Environmental Health II. D.D. Hemphill, Ed. pp. 7–27. University of Missouri Press, Columbia.

WHO Environmental Health Criteria 3: Lead. 1977. World Health Organization, Geneva.

Yamamoto, T., Yamaguchi, M. and Sato, H. 1975. Effects of cadmium acetate on bone acid hydrolase activity in rats treated with lead acetate. Eisei Kaguku 21:289–293.

6. Exposure to Lead

Paul B. Hammond

Natural Lead Exposure

It is impossible and probably unnecessary to eliminate lead totally from the human environment because it is a natural constituent of the earth's crust, just as are all the other elements. Rocks formed before man's existence contain approximately 13 μg Pb/g. Most soils have a very similar concentration. It has been suggested nonetheless that a very general pollution of man's environment has resulted from the introduction of lead for various purposes during and since the Industrial Revolution. The generalized nature of this pollution is based largely on evidence of lead contamination of glacial strata of recent date compared to strata formed many hundreds of years ago. It is very difficult to estimate what the consequences of this generalized pollution have been in terms of human contamination. Two approaches have been taken to evaluate this question: 1) comparison of the lead content of human bones antedating the Industrial Revolution with that of contemporary bones and 2) comparison of blood lead concentrations in various contemporary civilizations relative to lead exposure. These studies have been beset with numerous confounding variables which make interpretation extremely difficult. Even if all the evidence were clearly indicative of human contamination as a result of generalized pollution, the health consequences still would not be known.

Table 1.   Dietary intake of lead at various ages in young children (adapted from Mahaffey, 1976).

Age (mos)	μgPb/d	Assumed Weight (kg)	μgPb/kg
12–23	75.7	11	6.9
24–35	84.2	13.5	6.2
36–47	120.5	16	7.5

Normal Lead Exposure

The lead exposure of the child in utero is determined by the exposure of his mother. Indeed, there is a close correspondence between maternal blood lead concentration (PbB) and that of the child at birth, with the latter being higher by a factor of approximately 1.3, as indicated by analysis of umbilical cord PbB. The somewhat higher value of the newborn may possibly be explained on the basis of the higher hematocrit of newborns, since most of the lead in blood is localized in the erythrocytes.

During the first year of life lead exposure of the child is largely limited to air, food and beverages. In the normal situation these continue to be the usual sources of lead exposure during the remainder of childhood. The amount of lead in the diet is thought to be the major source of input. Because food consumption is more proportional to surface area than to body weight, dietary consumption of lead per unit body weight decreases as the child grows. Thus, in children less than 2 yr, dietary consumption of lead is approximately 10 μg/kg/day (Ziegler et al., 1978). In contrast, dietary lead intake in adulthood is probably only about 2 to 3 μg/kg/day. In normal children ages 2 to 6, dietary lead intake is probably about 4 to 8 μg/kg/day. These figures are derived from direct estimates of food consumption and from measurement of fecal lead excretion. The former approach assumes representativeness of the diets selected for lead analysis and the latter approach relies on the validity of the assumption that fractional absorption of ingested lead before it appears in the feces is 50%. In spite of these problems, the two approaches produce fairly consistent estimates of lead intake. Dr. Mahaffey and her colleagues (1976) have reported dietary lead intake for children with PbB <30 μg/dl (Table 1). The diets were self-selected. In a study conducted at the University of Cincinnati about the same time, long-term fecal lead excretion was measured in children with normal PbB living in homes free of lead paint (Hammond et al., 1980). The data are summarized in Table 2.

Table 2.   Fecal lead excretion in normal children (adapted from Hammond et al., 1980).

Subject	PbB	Collection Days	Fecal Pb Excretion (μg/kg/day)	Intake (μgPb/kg/day), Assuming 50% Absorption
1	18	19	4.6	9.2
2	15	14	2.9	5.8
		13	2.0	4.0
		14	1.7	3.4
		11	1.4	2.8
3	12	13	2.8	5.6

The other significant source of normal lead exposure in children is inhalation of ambient air. Although this exposure cannot be discounted completely, its impact is minor. Referring back to the relationship of blood lead to air lead (PbB/PbA) described in the previous discussion of lead metabolism (Chapter 2), it seems that even at 1 μgPb/m^3, a rather high value for normal ambient air, the contribution of air to PbB is unlikely to be more than 2.5 μg/day. The U.S. Environmental Protection Agency (EPA) estimates that the geometric mean PbB for children is approximately 12 μg/dl, excluding air sources. It has estimated that with an additional 1.5 μg/m^3 air lead level (the new air lead standard), PbB would be 15 μg/dl on the average and would stay below 30 μg/dl in more than 99% of children. This, then, is the current perception of normal lead exposure.

Abnormal Lead Exposure

It is generally agreed that the major concern today is excessive exposure of children in the inner cities. In the period 1930 to 1960 it became rather widely known that children with lead poisoning generally lived in houses where cracking and peeling paint was common. This, combined with the knowledge that children mouth, chew and swallow foreign objects, including paint chips, resulted in a general impression that lead-based paint was probably the major cause of pediatric lead poisoning. Other sources of lead were generally considered rather rare, e.g., fumes from burning battery casings. In 1972 the National Academy of Science published a review entitled "Airborne Lead in Perspective" to provide a scientific basis for development of criteria for setting limits for lead in ambient air (National Academy of Science, 1972). The document noted that city street dust and soil in the vicinity of freeways often had lead concentrations in excess of 1000 ppm. It was suggested that this might be a significant source of lead, caused principally by fallout from combusted lead in gasoline.

In the meantime, federally-sponsored lead screening programs were established to identify children with excessive lead exposure. City health departments publicized the hazards of lead and instituted abatement programs. Although the incidence of clinical lead poisoning fell dramatically during the late 1960's and early 1970's, elevated lead exposure of lesser magnitude persists.

Since 1972, numerous studies have been focused on the significance of lead in street dust and house dust (See Charney, Chapter 8.) In many instances it has been shown that children with elevated PbB live in houses free of lead paint, thereby putting the onus on hand-to-mouth transfer of lead-laden dust. Other studies have suggested a high correlation between traffic density and PbB, again suggesting fallout of lead from gasoline combustion as the cause. Unfortunately, the correlation between traffic density and fallout of lead in soil is very poor

(Johnson et al., 1978). Moreover, all these studies have assumed that PbB reflects the hazard of the current environment of the child. This assumption is valid only if the child has resided in his environment long enough for his PbB to reflect with reasonable accuracy the intake from his environment. As was pointed out in the discussion of lead metabolism (Chapter 2), PbB equilibrates only very slowly with lead intake. If a child moves from an environment where lead intake is high to one where lead intake is low, his PbB will remain high for months in spite of drastically reduced lead intake. As it happens, inner city families do move frequently. When this is the case, it is difficult to draw any conclusions about the hazards of a home environment based on PbB. By contrast, fecal lead excretion (PbF) does reflect current lead intake. This is dramatically evident in the case of two children with grossly elevated PbB who moved from a home environment which was highly hazardous with reference to lead-based paint to a low-hazard home environment (Hammond, 1980). PbF in these two children was determined for 9 days prior to and 9 days following the move. Average PbF was then determined repeatedly during the succeeding 20 months with fecal collection periods of 16 to 24 successive days. PbB was also determined periodically. The results are displayed graphically in Figure 1.

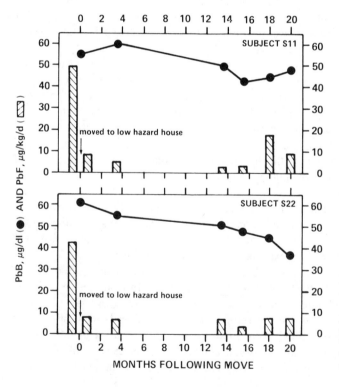

Fig. 1. Effect of moving from high hazard home to nearby low hazard home on PbB and PbF (Hammond et al., 1980. Reprinted with permission of *International Archives of Occupational and Environmental Health.*)

Table 3.   Long term fecal lead excretion in children (μg Pb/kg/day).

Collection Days	PbB	PbF, μg Pb/kg/day					
		Median	Mean	Four Highest Values			
19	70	8	9	11	15	15	17
13	21	8	14	13	16	23	76
13	48	16	16	24	29	32	34
12	69	6	8	12	13	19	21
8	73	9	17	12	12	17	76
13	60	4	4	6	6	10	11
22	53	14	150	47	58	190	2711
20	52	17	17	25	26	28	28
21	70	10	12	16	20	23	31
19	18	4	5	6	7	8	8
14	15	3	2	5	6	9	7
12	13	3	2	4	4	4	6

In the same study PbF was characterized in a number of children with elevated PbB who lived in houses with lead-based paint hazard. These data are summarized in Table 3. Note that the data for the last three children are quite different from those of the others. These children had normal PbB and lived in low-hazard houses. Both their median and mean PbF were considerably lower. Moreover, their PbF was much less variable, as reflected in the modest increases in PbF for the four highest days. These data suggest that children with high PbB engage in two general types of excessive lead ingestion, regular (elevated median PbF) and irregular (occasional grossly elevated PbF). The former is compatible with frequent hand-to-mouth transfer of house dust and the latter is compatible with eating small particles of lead-based paint.

If the household dust hypothesis is correct, it still remains to be established that lead-based paint is the source. The source of lead in dust may be essentially the same in all homes. The significant variables may be the amount of dust accumulation and the degree of child supervision. Mothers living in dilapidated housing may simply do less housecleaning than mothers in well maintained houses. In one recent study it was found that fecal lead excretion in children was not elevated in spite of the fact that fallout lead in soil was quite high in the vicinity of the residences (673 to 3633 μg/g) (Johnson et al., 1975). The subjects were children of university students living near a freeway. Housecleaning and child supervision may simply have been better there than in inner cities.

Point sources of lead emission have resulted in elevated childhood lead exposure, principally among children living near primary or secondary lead smelters and storage battery manufacturing plants. As with the situation in inner cities, the dust problem comes to the fore. In the vicinity of smelters where air lead levels usually are only moderately elevated and where dust lead levels usually are grossly elevated, only young children experience substantial eleva-

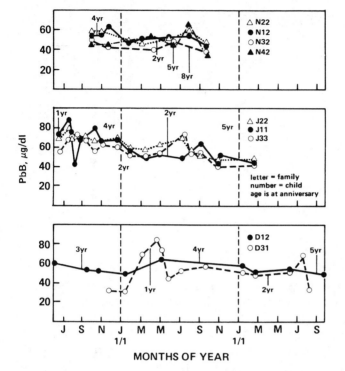

Fig. 2. Serial PbB levels in siblings of three families (Hammond et al., 1980. Reprinted with permission of *International Archives of Occupational and Environmental Health.*)

tion of PbB (Landrigan et al., 1975; Yankel and Von Lindern, 1977). This is highly suggestive of hand-to-mouth transfer.

The children of men working in lead smelters or battery factories may be at special risk because their fathers may bring significant amounts of lead dust home on their clothing or shoes. The significance of this source is highly dependent on the nature of the industrial hygiene program i.e., whether showering and changing at the workplace, of clothing and shoes at the factory are required and enforced.

The tracing of sources of lead in the environment of a child requires an understanding of the social and environmental setting of the family. For example, a home environment may be relatively free of lead hazards, but the child may spend a good deal of time outside the home or at the home of a grandparent. Alternatively, the play area may be grossly contaminated from unusual sources, e.g., sandblasting of buildings in the area. There simply is no substitute for good detective work.

Finally, it should be noted that more often than not, siblings of a child with elevated PbB will show a similar degree of lead exposure. This is illustrated in Figure 2.

Summary

Under usual conditions the major source of lead in humans is the diet. Children consume more food and food-derived lead in proportion to body weight than do adults, about 6 μg Pb/kg/day for toddlers versus 2 to 3 μg/kg/day for adults. Excessive lead exposure in young children has long been felt to result primarily from pica for chips of flaking and cracking lead-based paint in old houses. The incidence of grossly elevated lead exposure has decreased in recent years. Evidence is growing that hand-to-mouth transfer of house dust may be the major source of the more moderate degree of excessive lead exposure commonly encountered today. The sources of lead in house dust are defined imprecisely.

References

Hammond, P.B., et al. 1981. Int Arch Occup Environ Hlth 46:191.

Johnson, D.E. et al. 1975. Levels of platinum, palladium, and lead in populations of Southern California. Environ. Health Perspect. 12:27–33.

Johnson, D.E. et al. 1978. Epidemiological studies of the effects of automobile traffic on blood lead levels. EPA-600/1-78-055 :187.

Landrigan, P.J. et al. 1975. Epidemic lead absorption near an ore smelter. New England J Med 292:123.

Mahaffey, K.R., 1976. Relationships between quantities of lead ingested and health effects of lead in humans. Report prepared April 22, 1976, Bureau of Foods, Food and Drug Administration.

National Academy of Sciences. 1972. Airborne Lead in Perspective. Nat. Acad. Sci., Washington, D.C.

Yankel, A.J. and Von Lindern, I.H. 1977. The Silver Valley lead study: the relationship between childhood blood lead levels and environmental exposure. J Air Pollution Control Assn 27:763.

Ziegler et al. 1978. Absorption and retention of lead by infants. Pediat Res 12:29–34.

7. Role of Nutrition in Prevention of Pediatric Lead Toxicity

Kathryn R. Mahaffey

The role of nutritional status in altering susceptibility to lead toxicity has been investigated since the 1920's. Several nutritional factors have been shown to influence susceptibility to lead toxicity in experimental animals (Mahaffey, 1980). Many dietary deficiencies can be produced under experimental conditions that are unlikely to occur naturally in human populations eating Western-type diets. In this chapter, nutritional problems are emphasized that both influence lead toxicity and are likely to occur clinically.

Most of the data on factors affecting susceptibility to lead toxicity have been obtained from studies with experimental animals (Table 1). There is always controversy over applying data from animal experiments to human conditions, although in the case of metals their metabolism is more similar than different among species. However, the quantity of the metal that produces an effect may differ widely among species. Frequently, animal data may be applied to humans on a qualitative but not on a quantitative basis. Interactions between lead and

Table 1. Sources of information on susceptibility to lead toxicity.

I. Animal Experiments
II. Human Studies
    A Epidemiology
        1. environmental surveys
        2. health assessment surveys
        3. dietary surveys
        4. clinical observations
    B Metabolic Balance Studies

Table 2.   Nutrients recognized in 1979 as influencing susceptibility to lead toxicity.

1. Overall quantity of food intake
2. Major nutrients—protein, fat
3. Minerals—calcium, iron, phosphorus, zinc, copper, selenium
4. Vitamins—vitamin D, ascorbic acid, vitamin E

many nutrients have been confirmed in several species; for example, increased susceptibility to lead toxicity produced by calcium deficiency has been shown in rats (Mahaffey et al., 1973; Quarterman and Morrisson, 1975), dogs (Calvery et al., 1938), pigs (Hsu et al., 1975) and horses (Willoughby et al., 1972). Observations on humans indicate that certain metabolic and nutritional factors increase susceptibility to lead toxicity.

Of the many factors influencing susceptibility to lead intoxication, this chapter is limited to the effects of age and nutritional factors (Table 2). Elsewhere in this book, Drs. Charney (Chapter 8) and O'Hara (Chapter 9), describe social and behavioral aspects of susceptibility to lead toxicity.

Age

It is well recognized that in the United States the vast majority of nonindustrial lead toxicity occurs in children. In the general population, an association also exists between age and blood lead levels (Fig. 1). These data were obtained during the second National Health and Nutrition Evaluation Survey, which is not yet completed. Therefore, Figure 1 contains only data from the portion of the population examined between 1976 and 1978 (Mahaffey et al., 1980). These data were obtained from analyses of blood samples collected from people selected as representative of the general population, i.e., they were not under suspicion of having higher than normal exposure to lead. Because this is a

Table 3.   Percentage of examinees having elevated blood lead concentrations. (Raw data from a portion of the Second Health and Nutrition Examination Survey (HANES II) conducted by the National Center for Health Statistics, 1976-1978 (Mahaffey et al., 1980).

Lead Concentration*	Total Subjects (%)	Age 6 mos–6 yr (%)
≥30	3.5	5.7
≥40	0.76	1.3
≥50	0.32	0.66

*μg/dl whole blood.

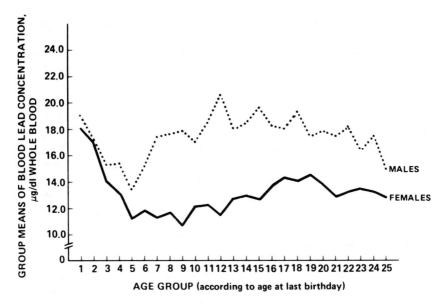

Fig. 1. Relationship between age and blood lead levels. Source, raw data from a portion of the Second Health and Nutrition Examination Survey (HANES II) conducted by the National Center for Health Statistics, 1976–1978 (Mahaffey et al., 1980).

preliminary report, the statistics presented in Table 1 are not national estimates. Rather, they show the overall distribution of lead levels among participants who reside in various communities across the United States and whose characteristics represent cross sections of socioeconomic and demographic strata. Age accounted for 15% of the variation in blood lead concentrations for persons 1 to 15 yr of age, while in juveniles and adults (16 to 74 yrs old), age accounted for only 1% of the variation in blood lead concentration. Table 3 presents the prevalence of examinees with blood lead concentrations greater than 30, 40 and 50 μg/dl of blood. Again it is emphasized that this population was selected as representative of persons having typical exposures to lead but that these data do not provide national estimates.

Several factors are involved in the higher prevalence of elevated blood lead concentrations in young children. Mouthing of objects or the presence of pica increases the quantity of lead ingested. In addition, young children absorb substantially more lead than adults. The results of two major metabolic balance studies of lead absorption in children are summarized in Table 4. Ziegler et al. (1978) observed that children absorb a much higher percentage of ingested lead than adults and that there is high individual variability in lead absorption among children. Adults in a nonfasting state usually absorb 5 to 10% of ingested lead; however, individual adults absorb between 1 and 15% of ingested lead. In the balance studies of Ziegler et al., infants, 14 to 746 days of age, were investigated for age-related differences in lead absorption. Differences in lead absorption between infants and toddlers were not observed in this study. These data apply only to levels of lead exposure higher than 5 μg/kg body weight per day. Below this level of lead exposure, children excreted more lead than they ingested from food.

A third metabolic balance study (Barltrop and Strehlow, 1978) found that young children were consistently in negative lead balance at levels of lead intake higher than 5 μg/kg body weight per day. Results of this study are quite difficult to associate with a much larger amount of information on lead metabolism. For example, it is well known that people accumulate an increasing body burden of lead as they age (Barry, 1978). If children were consistently in negative lead balance, this body burden of lead would be expected to decrease rather than increase.

Based on previous reports, it is likely that children absorb a higher percentage of ingested lead than do adults. It is prudent patient management to assume that, compared with adults, children absorb greater quantities of lead. Unfortunately, we do not know at what age childrens' absorption of lead changes to patterns seen in adults. For example, it is not clear if 6- or 8-yr-olds resemble adults more closely than they resemble 2-yr-olds with regard to lead absorption. Age is a variable that helps the physician identify patients at greater risk of developing lead toxicity but is not a factor that can be used to control susceptibility to lead toxicity.

Nutrition

Turning now to nutritional factors, there is a great deal of information indicating that nutritional status can influence susceptibility to lead toxicity (Mahaffey, 1980). Fortunately, nutritional status can be changed. The role of nutrition in management of patients at high risk of lead toxicity is preventive rather than therapeutic. In the 1930's and 1940's the use of diet to "delead" patients was evaluated. Chelation therapy (Hardy et al., 1954) has provided a far more successful method of mobilization of lead from the body, although it may produce nutritional problems in patients with severe lead intoxication due to removal of zinc and other trace elements from the patient. The role of nutritional intervention is to try to reduce absorption and tissue accumulation of body burden of lead in children known to be at high risk of elevated lead exposure. Although a number of nutritional factors alter susceptibility to lead intoxication at the cellular level, emphasis is given only to those nutrients that are known to be ingested in less than adequate quantities by portions of the general population.

Table 4.   Absorption and retention of lead by infants and children.

Investigator	Subjects	No.	Absorption (%)	Retention (%)
Alexander et al. (1972)	Healthy children, 3 mos to 8.5 yr; children with inborn errors of metabolism, 3 wk to 8.5 yr	8 children 6 children	50* 24†	18* 10†
Ziegler et al. (1978)	Normal infants 14–746 days	12 children, 89 balances	41.5‡	31.7‡

*Lead intake 10.6 μg/kg body weight/day (regular mixed diet).
†Lead intake 14.5 μg/kg body weight/day (synthetic diets, i.e., low phenylalanine, etc.).
‡When lead intake was greater than 5 μg Pb/kg body weight/day. Below this level of lead exposure, children excreted more lead than was ingested in the diet during the 3-day balance study period.

Several nutritional surveys have been carried out on children during the past 10 years; many of these surveys were reviewed by Owen and Lippman (1977). Some nutrients, for which nutritional status of the general population is not well known, are known to influence susceptibility to lead toxicity. Among these are vitamin E, selenium and copper. Under medical conditions requiring treatment such as hyperalimentation, deficiency or toxicity of many nutrients is a potential problem. This discussion, however, emphasizes nutritional problems, such as dietary deficiencies of iron, calcium, zinc and ascorbic acid, recognized to be prevalent in outpatients or in persons appearing clinically well, especially children.

Overall patterns of food intake influence absorption of lead. Data on five human subjects 25 to 53 years of age reported by Rabinowitz et al. (1975) showed that lead ingested between meals was absorbed to a far greater extent (70%) than was lead ingested with meals (6 to 14%). In a dietary survey among low income center city children living in Washington DC about 5 years ago, some of the dietary records indicated small food intakes for some children. Interviewers pointed out that the type and supply of food changed dramatically throughout the month in relation to the arrival of support payments, and that because of this it would be valuable to record the time of month in which the surveying was done. This situation may not exist generally, but the importance of balanced, regular patterns of food intake to minimize lead absorption must be considered.

Calcium is a nutrient known to be of importance in susceptibility to lead effects. Blood lead concentrations of rats exposed to identical quantities of lead are much higher in groups ingesting a low calcium diet than in groups receiving an adequate calcium diet (Fig. 2). Low calcium diets also facilitate accumulation

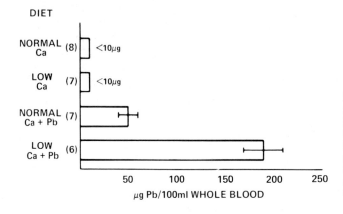

Fig. 2. Influence of dietary calcium on blood lead levels (Mahaffey-Six and Goyer, 1970. Reprinted with permission of the *Journal of Laboratory and Clinical Medicine.*)

of lead in the femur and the kidney (Table 5). Other indicators of lead toxicity, including urinary excretion of delta-aminolevulinic acid and development of renal intranuclear inclusion bodies (Mahaffey, 1974), reflect the influence of a low calcium diet on tissue accumulation of lead (Table 6). From dose-response studies in rats, Mahaffey et al. (1973) found that a low calcium diet increased susceptibility to lead toxicity approximately 20-fold. In all these experiments, the rats were exposed to identical quantities of lead; the differences in levels of lead in tissues and clinical indicators of lead toxicity were attributable to ingestion of a low calcium diet.

The mechanisms by which a low calcium diet increases susceptibility to lead toxicity are not fully known but include changes in absorption and tissue distribution of lead. Barton et al. (1978a), using rat intestine, observed that as the quantity of calcium in the intubation media was increased, lead absorption

Table 5.   Effect of dietary calcium deficiency on blood, kidney and femur Pb concentration in rats (Mahaffey-Six and Goyer, 1970. Reprinted with permission of the *Journal of Laboratory and Clinical Medicine.*)

Calcium Level	Kidney Pb, μg/g*	Femur Pb, μg/g*
Normal Ca[†]	2.6 ± 1.2[‡]	2.2 ± 1.0
Low Ca[§]	4.4 ± 0.6	9.7 ± 2.2
Normal Ca + Pb[‖]	29.6 ± 7.0	202.0 ± 22.2
Low Ca ± Pb	691.0 ± 203.0	225.0 ± 15.2

*Wet weight.
[†]0.7% of diet.
[‡]Mean ± SEM.
[§]0.1% of diet.
[‖]Pb in drinking water; 200 ppm Pb added as lead acetate.

Table 6. Minimal concentration of lead in drinking water of rats that produces various lead-induced changes (Mahaffey, 1974).

	Minimal Toxic Dose, μg Pb/ml	
Change	Low Calcium Diet*	Normal Calcium Diet†
Intranuclear inclusion bodies‡	12	200
Increased urinary excretion of delta-aminolevulinic acid	12	200
Increased kidney weight/body weight ratio	3	200

*0.1% Ca.
†0.7% Ca.
‡In renal proximal tubule lining cell.

declined (Fig. 3). Similar results were observed also for human subjects in the balance data of Ziegler et al. (1978) from infants and toddlers (Fig. 4). As calcium levels in the diet decreased, lead absorption increased. Results of studies on lead/calcium interactions in experimental animals indicate that the greatest increases in susceptibility to lead toxicity occurred with calcium-deficient diets. The human metabolic balance data are particularly impressive because all levels of calcium fed to the children met nutritional recommendations for calcium for children (Fomon, 1974).

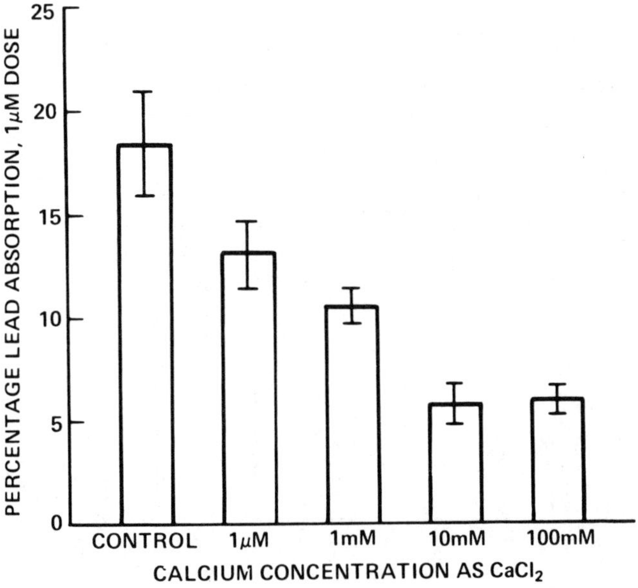

Fig. 3. Effect of variation of $CaCl_2$ in the intubation media on absorption of a single dose of radiolabeled $PbCl_2$ (Barton et al., 1978a. Reprinted with permission of the *Journal of Laboratory and Clinical Medicine.*)

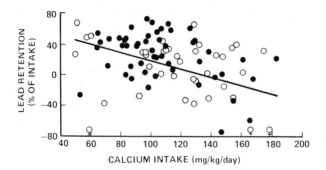

Fig. 4. Lead retention in relation to calcium intake (Ziegler et al., 1978. Reprinted with permission of *Pediatric Research.*)

Calcium also influences the release of lead stored in bone. Rosen and Wexler (1977) have demonstrated that, if the level of calcium in the culture media were lowered, rat bones under culture released greater quantities of lead than they did when the level of calcium was higher. Currently the role of dietary calcium in stimulating release of lead from bone has not been investigated in humans; however, it is reasonable to believe that this occurs. Clinical diagnosis of mild cases of calcium deficiency in humans is not simple and perhaps not possible with current techniques. Under conditions of adequate vitamin D intake and a functioning parathyroid gland, serum calcium will not change dramatically in a patient because the bone supplies a vast reservoir of calcium. However, in lead-exposed patients the bone also supplies a vast reservoir of lead. This emphasizes the importance of consistently supplying adequate dietary calcium, both to minimize lead absorption and to minimize resorption of calcium and lead from the bone.

Several dietary surveys (Sorrell et al., 1977; Mahaffey et al., 1976; Johnson and Tenuta, 1979) have evaluated nutrient intake among lead-burdened children

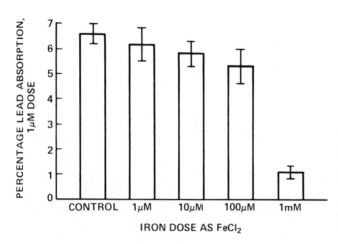

Fig. 5. Effect of variation of $FeCl_2$ in the intubation media on the absorption of radiolabeled $PbCl_2$ (Barton et al., 1978b. Reprinted with permission of the *Journal of Laboratory and Clinical Medicine.*)

Table 7.   Dietary calcium (mg/day) intake in control and lead-burdened children.

Investigator	Control Children	Lead-burdened Children
Mahaffey et al. (1976)	570 ± 23*	457 ± 18*
Sorrell et al. (1977)	800 ± 30*	580 ± 15*
Johnson and Tenuta (1979)	615 ± 245†	468 ± 152†

*Mean ± 1 SEM.
†Mean ± 1 SD.

and matched control children (Table 7). Consistently, these studies have shown a lower dietary calcium intake among children with elevated body stores of lead. The Ten-State Nutrition Survey 1968-1970 (1972A) investigated dietary calcium intake among low income children. The percentage distribution of children ingesting various levels of calcium in their diets is shown in Table 8.

Table 8.   Cumulative percentage distribution of calcium and iron intakes for children 24 to 36 mos of age for low income ratio states (data are from the 10-State Nutrition Survey, 1968-1970, 1972a).

Calcium		Iron	
Intake (mg/day)	Children (%)	Intake (mg/day)	Children (%)
200	13.7	3.9	24.1
400	28.9	7.9	67.3
600	50.1	11.9	90.9
800*	65.9	15.0*	98.0

*Recommended dietary allowances for children 2 to 3 yr old (National Research Council, 1974).

Phosphorus, like calcium, is a nutrient that affects lead metabolism (Quarterman and Morrison, 1975). Phosphorus deficiency will increase susceptibility to lead toxicity. However, Western-type diets are usually quite high in phosphorus so that no special attention is required to maintain an adequate intake of this nutrient.

The clinical situation with iron is quite different from that of phosphorus. Iron deficiency and iron deficiency anemia are the most common nutritional deficiencies in the United States (Woodruff, 1977). Owen et al. (1971) studied 3423 preschool children from impoverished to upper middle income groups and found that approximately 5% of the children had iron deficiency anemia (defined as a hemoglobin concentration of less than 10 g/dl in children between 1 and 2 yr of age and less than 11 grams/dl in children between 2 and 6 yr) and that prevalence was negatively associated with socioeconomic status. Iron deficiency is known to increase susceptibility to lead toxicity in rats. Table 9 shows the effect of a low iron diet on tissue accumulation of lead in rats (Mahaffey et al., 1978). It is important to emphasize that these rats had mild, not severe, iron deficiency. By

Table 9.   Influence of dietary iron on susceptibility to lead toxicity in rats (Mahaffey et al., 1978).

| | Low Pb Exposure* | | |
Dietary Fe	Blood Pb ug/dl	Kidney Pb ppm	Femur Pb ppm
Deficient (10 ppm)	5.9 ± 0.05‡	1.3 ± 0.18	3.11 ± 0.26‡
Adequate (40 ppm)	9.7 ± 1.8	1.05 ± 0.14	1.04 ± 0.14
High (120 ppm)	5.8 ± 1.0	0.85 ± 0.10	5.8 ± 1.0

*Deionized water, diet <0.01 ppm Pb.
‡Mean ± SEM.

analogy to humans this is not the severe form of iron deficiency that is associated with a hemoglobin concentration of 5 or 6 g/dl of blood, but the degree of iron deficiency that is associated with a hemoglobin concentration of 11 g/dl and reduced serum iron. Table 10 presents the percentage distribution of children having less than 15% transferrin saturation; if transferrin saturation is less than 15%, the iron supply to the bone marrow is considered inadequate (Owen et al., 1971).

Mahaffey et al. (1978) demonstrated that tissue lead levels were reduced if rats were fed diets containing iron at levels above those recommended on a nutritional basis. As is the situation with calcium, very little is known about the mechanism(s) by which iron deficiency increases susceptibility to lead toxicity. Iron deficiency increases absorption of lead from the gastrointestinal tract. Barton et al. (1978b) measured lead absorption in rats and found that increased concentrations of iron in the intubation media decreased lead absorption (Fig. 5). Varying the dietary levels of iron appears to affect absorption of lead rather than lead excretion. Barton et al. (1978b) measured lead excretion by rats which

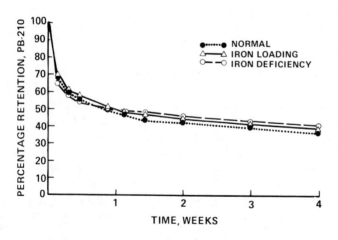

Fig. 6. Comparison of the retention of ^{210}Pb by normal, iron-loaded and iron-deficient rats (Barton et al., 1978b. Reprinted with permission of the *Journal of Laboratory and Clinical Medicine.*)

High Pb Exposure[†]		
Blood Pb ug/dl	Kidney Pb ppm	Femur Pb ppm
159 ± 8	311 (254,382)§	339 ± 14
113 ± 11	44 (33,61)	209 ± 22
76 ± 7	26 (19,36)	187 ± 23

[†]200 ppm Pb in water, diet <0.01 ppm Pb.
§Data log transformed, error estimates not symmetrical about the mean.

either were iron-deficient, had normal body stores of iron or were iron-loaded. The data shown in Figure 6 demonstrate that iron status did not influence the excretion of lead. Clinically, this means that iron prevents the accumulation of body burden of lead rather than stimulating excretion of lead. These studies by Barton et al. are useful in interpreting the report by Angle et al. (1976) on iron therapy for lead-burdened children. The latter investigators observed that administration of oral iron therapy did not lower blood lead concentrations among children exposed to lead. However, the subjects had elevated blood lead concentrations at the start of their therapeutic programs. If this study is viewed with the knowledge that iron status does not alter lead excretion, then the negative findings of Angle et al. are understandable.

Some of the types of data that are available to establish the effects of dietary calcium level on lead metabolism do not yet exist for iron. For example, metabolic balance data on lead absorption by iron-deficient children are not yet

Table 10. Percentage distribution of reduced transferrin saturation* by age and socioeconomic status[†] (Owen et al., 1971).

Age (mos)	Socioeconomic Status	Children with Transferrin Saturation <15% (%)
12—23	I	68
	II	52
	III	35
	IV	39
24—33	I	37
	II	29
	III	21
	IV	18
36—47	I	36
	II	24
	III	27
	IV	18

*Serum Iron/total serum iron binding capacity × 100.
[†]Index stratification characteristics (% of families in each ranking): I, lower, lower (18%); II, upper, lower (40%); III, lower, middle (31%); IV, upper, middle (11%) (Warner, 1960).

available. Further, dietary surveys have not shown a clear reduction in dietary iron intake among lead-burdened children.

Zinc is another trace element important in susceptibility to lead toxicity. Zinc deficiency is known to increase tissue lead levels in animals exposed to equal doses of lead (Cerklewski and Forbes, 1976). Further, zinc at the cellular level protects some enzymes required for heme synthesis against the effects of lead. For example, the activity of delta-aminolevulinic acid dehydratase in animals is inhibited by lead (Meredith et al., 1974), but the degree of inhibition can be greatly reduced by increasing the amount of zinc fed to them (Finelli et al., 1975). Zinc deficiency has been demonstrated clinically in humans. Among low income preschool children in Denver, two-thirds of the subjects had low concentrations of zinc in the hair and serum (Hambidge, 1977).

In addition to changes in susceptibility to lead toxicity produced by trace elements, two major nutrients are also of importance in altering susceptibility to lead toxicity: protein and fat. Diets containing moderate or normal amounts of protein have been shown to be the most beneficial in terms of susceptibility to lead toxicity; with low or high protein diets increasing the severity of effects of lead exposure (Baernstein and Grand, 1942; Gontzea et al., 1964; Barltrop and Khoo, 1975). Some amino acids facilitate lead absorption (Barton et al., 1978b), which might explain the increased effects of lead that occur when a high protein diet is fed.

A similar picture exists for dietary fat. Barltrop and Khoo (1975) have shown in rats that high fat diets facilitate lead absorption and increase tissue lead concentrations (Table 11). Reducing the dietary fat level to nearly zero did not reduce lead concentrations in tissues. It is very difficult to translate this data to humans on a quantitative basis because rats normally consume a diet much lower in fat than do humans. In terms of human nutrition, the diet typically consumed by people in the United States is much higher in fat than is required nutritionally; many nutritional and medical authorities have recommended a restricted fat intake for a number of reasons unrelated to lead. Regarding susceptibility to lead toxicity, the important finding from the work of Barltrop and Khoo is that high fat diets produce elevated tissue lead concentrations.

The role of vitamins in relation to lead toxicity is complicated. In time we may discover that lead has a greater effect on the metabolism of vitamins than vitamins have on the metabolism of lead, but conclusive information in this area is still not available. Vitamin D has been associated with susceptibility to lead toxicity, possibly because of the higher incidence of lead toxicity in the summer and possibly because of the effects of vitamin D on calcium and phosphorus metabolism. Smith et al. (1978) have shown that vitamin D stimulated lead absorption in vitamin D-deprived animals. Increasing vitamin D administration above physiologic levels did not increase the rats' lead absorption above that observed when vitamin D was fed at the physiologic requirement for the vitamin. Mahaffey et al. (1979) reported that 1,25-dihydroxycholecalciferol was the form

Table 11.   Effect of dietary fat on blood, kidney and femur lead concentration* in rats (Barltrop and Khoo, 1975).

Dietary Fat (%)	Blood	Kidney	Femur
Low, 0	1	1	1
Normal, 5	1	1	1
High, 40	9.6	7.6	4.8

*Ratio of mean retention experimental:control.

of vitamin D that stimulated absorption of lead. Rosen et al. (1980) have observed that lead-burdened children have reduced ability to form the active metabolite of vitamin D even though their dietary intake of vitamin D was normal, as shown by serum levels of 25-hydroxycholecalciferol. Based on current knowledge of the interactions of lead and vitamin D, changing vitamin D levels in the diets of patients would be inadvisable since vitamin D is a required nutrient and is needed for absorption of essential mineral nutrients such as calcium. High levels of vitamin D are inadvisable also, as too high an intake can produce vitamin D toxicity, specifically soft tissue calcification.

A similar set of circumstances exists for ascorbic acid. Lowering the level of ascorbic acid in the diet is inadvisable because vitamin C is an essential nutrient. High dietary levels of ascorbic acid did not alter tissue lead concentrations in guinea pigs fed ten times the recommended level of vitamin C (Mahaffey and Banks, 1974). Vitamin E deficiency greatly increased the susceptibility of rats to lead toxicity (Levander et al., 1975 and 1977a), particularly increasing red blood cell fragility (Levander et al., 1977b) and severity of lead-induced anemia. In humans, vitamin E deficiency is not considered prevalent in the pediatric population. However, very few dietary surveys have attempted to establish vitamin E status in children, so that complete clinical evaluation of this interaction cannot be made at this time.

An appropriate diet can increase resistance to lead toxicity, again emphasizing that the role of nutrition is to minimize accumulation of lead rather than to reduce a previously accumulated body burden of lead. The role of nutrition is in preventive medicine rather than treatment of acute lead intoxication. Important dietary principles include the following.

1. Attempt to provide regular balanced food intake.
2. Provide quantities of zinc and calcium at levels that are recommended by nutritional authorities such as the National Research Council (1978).
3. Do not provide high levels of mineral supplements. Although deficiency of a nutrient may increase susceptibility to lead toxicity, high levels of supplementation may also increase susceptibility. If the levels of these nutritional supplements are high enough, they may be toxic in themselves.

4. Be aware that there is some evidence that higher levels of iron than are now recommended by nutritionists may be useful in preventing lead toxicity. Children may require iron supplements if their eating patterns do not provide enough iron in food.

5. Plan diets to contain levels in vitamins in accordance with recommendations by nutritional authorities, such as the National Research Council's Recommended Dietary Allowances (1978). Avoid diets or supplements containing high levels of vitamins because some vitamins are toxic when consumed at high levels and there is no evidence that these are beneficial for prevention of lead toxicity.

In providing dietary advice to specific patients, certain family abilities and preferences should be considered. First of all, the family must be able to afford the diet. There are a variety of federal food programs, such as food stamps or the Special Supplemental Food Program for Women, Infants and Children, that help low income families pay for food. A dietitian or health department personnel can advise physicians or other responsible persons on the programs available in their community. Egan (1977) described the types of federal food programs that are available.

In addition, the child must like the diet. In part, this means that the diet must be suitable for the ethnic, regional and cultural background of the child and his family (USDHEW, 1972b). Food habits common to young children should also be considered. For example, many 2- and 3-yr-olds reject meat, particularly lean red meats that provide good sources of iron, zinc, and protein.

Finally, the diet preparation must be within the ability of the family. Familial factors such as working mothers, limited cooking and food storage facilities and limited food preparation abilities restrict the types of food or menus that should be suggested.

Physicians are required to use a great deal of information when treating patients; extensive knowledge of food composition is usually not their specialized knowledge. However, with the above general guidelines, a dietitian should be able to help the families of children and their physicians select diets to lower the risk of the child of accumulating undue body burdens of lead.

In Chapter 9, O'Hara describes the social aspects of susceptibility to lead toxicity. Some of these social factors also influence the likelihood of children receiving nutritionally adequate diets. The economic level of the family may be associated with an increased likelihood of living in a high lead environment. Children from low income families are also at greater risk of nutritional deficiencies, such as iron deficiency, than do other children. The coexistence of these circumstances means that the child is at greater risk of lead toxicity than if either circumstance occurred alone.

Improvement of nutritional status and control of environmental exposure to lead should be seen as separate public health goals. Ideally, standards on environmental exposure to lead should protect nutritionally deprived persons as well as individuals having optimal nutritional status. However, the effectiveness of environmental lead control can be optimized if children are well nourished.

References

Alexander, F.W., Clayton, B.F. and Delves, H.T. 1972. The uptake and excretion by children of lead and other contaminants. In Environmental Health Aspects of Lead. Commission of the European Communities, Luxembourg.

Angle, C.R., Stelmark, K.L. and McIntire, M.S. 1976. Lead and iron deficiency. In Trace Substances in Environmental Health, X. Hemphill, H.H., Ed. University of Missouri Press, Columbia.

Baernstein, H.D. and Grand, J.A. 1942. The relation of protein intake to lead poisoning in rats. J Pharmacol Exp Ther 4:18.

Barltrop, D. and Khoo, H.E. 1975. The influence of nutritional factors on lead absorption. Postgrad Md J 51:795.

Barltrop, D. and Stehlow, C.D. 1978. The absorption of lead by children. In Trace Element Metabolism in Man and Animals-3. Kirchgessner, M., Ed. Arbeitskreis für Tierernährungsforschung Weihenstephan, Freising-Weihenstephan, West Germany, pp. 332–334.

Barry, P.S.I. 1978. Distribution and storage of lead in human tissue. In Biogeochemistry of Lead in the Environment. Nriagu, O., Ed. Elsevier/North Holland Biomedical Press, Amsterdam.

Barton, J.C., Conrad, M.E., Harrison, L. and Nuby, S. 1978a. Effects of calcium on the absorption and retention of lead. J Lab Clin Med 91:367.

Barton, J.C., Conrad, M.E., Nuby, S. and Harrison, L. 1978b. Effect of iron on the absorption and retention of lead. J Lab Clin Med 92:536.

Calvery, H.O., Laug, E.P. and Morris, H.J. 1938. The chronic effects on dogs of feeding diets containing lead acetate, lead arsenate and arsenic trioxide in varying concentrations. J Pharmacol Exp Ther 64:365.

Cerklewski, F.L. and Forbes, R.M. 1976. The influence of dietary zinc on lead toxicity in the rat. J Nutr 106:689.

Egan, M.G. 1977. Federal nutrition support programs for children. Pediatr Clin North Am 24:229.

Finelli, V.N., Klauder, D.S., Karaffa, M.A. and Petering, H.G. 1975. Interaction of zinc and lead on delta-aminolevulinate dehydratase. Biochem Biophys Res Commun 65:303.

Fomon, S.J. 1974. Infant Nutrition. W.B. Saunders and Co., Philadelphia.

Gontzea, I., Sutzesco, P., Cocora, D. and Lungu, D. 1964. Importance de rapport de proteins sur las resistance del l'organisme a l'intoxication par le plomb. Arch Sci Physiol 18:211.

Hambidge, K.M. 1977. The role of zinc and other trace metals in pediatric nutrition and health. Pediatr Clin North Am 24:95.

Hardy, H.L., Elkins, H.B., Ruotolo, B.P., Quinby, J. and Baker, W.H. 1954. Use of monocalcium disodium ethylene diamine tetra-acetic acid in lead poisoning. J Am Med Assoc 154:1171.

Hsu, F.S., Krook, L., Pond, W.G. and Duncan, J.R. 1975. Interaction of dietary calcium with toxic levels of lead and zinc in pigs. J Nutr 105:112.

Johnson, N.E. and Tenuta, K. 1979. Zinc, iron and calcium intakes of lead poisoned children who practice pica. Environ Res 18:369.

Levander, O.A., Fisher, M., Morris, V.C. and Ferretti, R.J. (1977a). Morphology of erythrocytes from vitamin E-deficient lead-poisoned rats. J Nutr 107:1828.

Levander, O.A., Morris, V.C. and Ferretti, R.J. (1977b). Comparative effects of selenium and vitamin E in lead-poisoned rats. J Nutr 107:378.

Levander, O.A., Morris, V.C., Higgs, D.J. and Ferretti, R.J. 1975. Lead poisoning in vitamin E-deficient rats. J Nutr 105:1481.

Mahaffey, K.R. 1974. Nutritional factors and susceptibility to lead toxicity. Environ Health Perspect 7:107.

Mahaffey, K.R. 1980. Nutrient-lead interactions. In Lead Toxicity. Singhal, R. and Thomas, J.A., Eds. Urban and Schwarzenberg, Baltimore.

Mahaffey, K.R., Annest, L., Barbanos, H. and Murphy, R.S. 1980. Preliminary analysis of blood lead concentrations for children and adults: HANES II, 1976–1978. In Trace Substances in Environmental Health, XII. Hemphill, H.H., Ed. University of Missouri Press, Columbia. pp. 37–51.

Mahaffey, K.R. and Banks, T.A. 1974. Effect of varying dietary ascorbic acid on lead toxicity in guinea pigs. Fed Proc 32:267.

Mahaffey, K.R., Goyer, R.A. and Haseman, J. 1973. Dose-response to lead ingestion in rats on low dietary calcium. J Lab Clin Med 82:92.

Mahaffey, K.R., Smith, C., Tanaka, Y. and DeLuca, H.F. 1979. Stimulation of lead absorption by various vitamin D metabolites. Fed Proc 38:384.

Mahaffey, K.R., Stone, C.L., Banks, T.A. and Reed, G. 1978. Reduction in tissue storage of lead in the rat by feeding diets with elevated iron concentration. In Trace Element Metabolism in Man and Animals-3. Kirchgessner, M., Ed. Arbeitskreis für Tierernährungsforschung Weihenstephen, Freising-Weihenstephen, West Germany. pp. 584–588.

Mahaffey, K.R., Treloar, S., Banks, T.A., Peacock, B.J. and Parekh, L.E. 1976. Differences in dietary intake of calcium and phosphorus in children having normal and elevated blood lead concentrations. J Nutr 106:xxx (abstract).

Mahaffey-Six, K. and Goyer, R.A. 1970. Experimental enhancement of lead toxicity by low dietary calcium. J Lab Clin Med 76:933.

Meredith, P.A., Moore, M.R. and Goldberg, A. 1974. The effects of aluminum, lead and zinc on delta-aminolevulinic acid dehydratase. Biochem Soc Trans 2:1243.

National Research Council, National Academy of Sciences 1974. Recommended Dietary Allowances, National Academy of Sciences, Washington.

National Research Council, National Academy of Sciences 1978. Recommended Dietary Allowances, National Academy of Sciences, Washington.

Owen, G. and Lippman, G. 1977. Nutritional status of infants and young children: U.S.A.

Pediatr Clin North Am 24:211.

Owen, G., Lubin, A.H. and Garry, P.J. 1971. Preschool children in the United States: Who has iron deficiency? J Pediatr 79:563.

Quarterman, J. and Morrison, J.N. 1975. The effects of dietary calcium and phosphorus on the retention and excretion of lead in rats. Br J Nutr 34:351.

Rabinowitz, M., Wetherill, G. and Kopple, J. 1975. Absorption, storage and excretion of lead by normal humans. In Trace Substances in Environmental Health, IX. Hemphill, H.H., Ed. University of Missouri Press, Columbia. p. 361.

Rosen, J.F., Chesney, R.W., Hamstra, A., DeLuca, H.F. and Mahaffey, K.R. 1980. Reduction of 1,25-dihydroxyvitamin D in children with increased lead absorption. N Engl J Med 302:1128.

Rosen, J.F., and Wexler, E.E. 1977. Studies of lead transport in bone organ culture. Biochem. Pharmacol. 26:650.

Smith, C.M., DeLuca, H.F., Tanaka, Y. and Mahaffey, K.R. 1978. Stimulation of lead absorption by vitamin D administration. J Nutr 108:843.

Sorrell, M., Rosen, J.F. and Roginsky, M.R. 1977. Interactions of lead, calcium, vitamin D and nutrition in lead-burdened children. Arch Environ Health 32:160.

USDHEW 1972a. Ten-State Nutrition Survey, 1968-1970. V. Dietary. Atlanta.

USDHEW 1972b. Practices of Low-income Families in Feeding Infants and Small Children. Proceedings of a conference. Health Services and Mental Health Administration, Maternal and Child Health Service, Rockville.

Warner, W.L. 1960. Social Class in America. Harper and Row, New York. pp. 149–150.

Willoughby, R.A., Triapatsakun, T. and McSherry, B.J. 1972. Influence of rations low in calcium and phosphorus on blood and tissue lead concentrations in the horse. Am J Vet Res 33:1165.

Woodruff, C.W. 1977. Iron deficiency in infancy and childhood. Pediatr Clin North Am 24:85.

Ziegler, E.E., Edwards, B.B., Jensen, R.L., Mahaffey, K.R. and Fomon, S.J. 1978. Absorption and retention of lead by infants. Pediatr Res 12:29.

8. Lead Poisoning in Children: The Case Against Household Lead Dust

Evan Charney

This chapter considers the source and mechanism of lead ingestion in urban children with subencephalopathic lead poisoning. We present recent work by Dr. James Sayre and myself to explore one specific hypothesis, that lead-containing household dust is a major source of lead for these children, with hand contamination and repetitive mouthing the proposed mechanism of ingestion. A series of studies that address this issue will be discussed.

Although frank lead encephalopathy has become uncommon in the United States, large numbers of children still show evidence of an increased body lead burden. For example, for the fiscal year 1979, 32,500 high risk children screened had blood lead (PbB) values in excess of 30 μg/dl (Morbidity and Mortality Weekly Report, 1980). The exact source of this lead exposure has not been clearly defined for the majority of these children. Repetitive swallowing of lead-contaminated paint chips probably accounts for most overtly symptomatic cases, but has been questioned as the principal source for those with mild to moderately elevated levels (Class II or III by USPHS standards).

We became concerned about the source of lead poisoning in the course of reviewing data from a 1971 prevalence study conducted in Rochester, New York. In that study blood lead levels were determined on 171 inner city children between 1 and 6 years of age who lived in the "lead belt" of the city. The children were selected in a door-to-door survey; although none showed evidence of central nervous system toxicity, the relatively high mean PbB value for the group (44 μg/dl) suggested a surprisingly widespread intake of lead. Routine testing of an additional 488 children living in the same area over the subsequent year showed a similar distribution of PbB values. Blood drawn from 51 adults

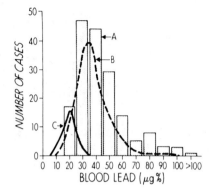

Fig. 1. Blood lead levels in three Rochester, New York, surveys (A. random sample, 1971, N = 171; B. Follow-up sample, 1972, N = 488; C. inner city adults, N = 51).

living in the same area showed substantially lower levels (mean PbB, 20 μg/dl), as did PbB from a sample of suburban Rochester children (mean PbB, 22 μg/dl). These data are shown in Figure 1. The nature of the distribution curve suggested a ubiquitous but low level source of lead exposure affecting a large number of city children, but sparing both adults in the same environment and suburban children. Drinking water and air lead levels were quite low and there were no known industrial sources of pollution in the study area.

While obtaining simultaneous capillary and venous specimens for PbB analysis, it was noted that the children's hands contained a quantity of lead sufficient to elevate markedly the finger capillary values unless their hands were scrupulously cleaned. We speculated that this might be an important clue; the mechanism of poisoning might involve hand contamination by repeated contact with floors and window sills in the environment and subsequent ingestion by the frequent hand-to-mouth activities of preschool children. To explore that hypothesis further, the amount of lead in household dust and on the hands of children in city and suburban homes was compared (Sayre et al., 1974). Fifty-one inner city and 51 suburban children between 9 mos and 6 years of age were selected for study. The amount of lead on the hands of the children was determined by thoroughly rubbing both hands with a paper towel (14 by 20 cm) impregnated with 20% denatured alcohol and benzalkonium chloride. Towel wipe specimens were also taken from an interior window sill surface and from a 1-ft sq uncarpeted floor area in the home where the child commonly played. This technique of determining the absolute quantity of Pb in a defined area, i.e., hands, a window sill and an area of floor, was selected in preference to assessing concentration of lead in the specimen. The critical factor in childhood lead poisoning is the amount of lead ingested, and that value is more accurately reflected by the total quantity of lead than it is by the concentration of lead in a sample. Lead content of the paper towel was determined by soaking the towel in 0.1 N hydrochloric

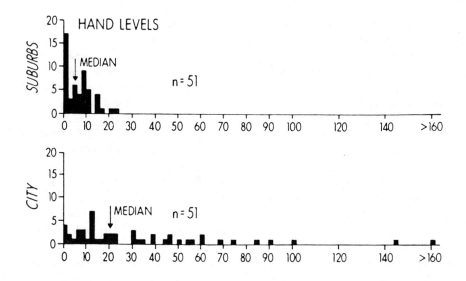

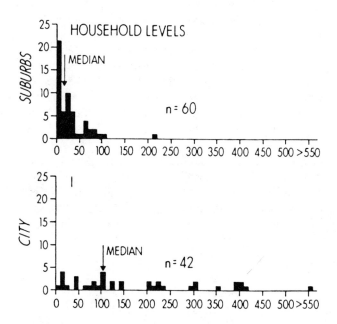

Fig. 2. Amount of lead on the hands of children and in household dust of inner city versus suburban homes. At top, horizontal axis: μg lead on hands of inner city and suburban children; vertical axis: number of patients. At bottom, horizontal axis: μg lead on household surfaces (windowsill or 0.09-sq m floor area) of inner city and suburban homes; vertical axis: number of specimens (Sayre et al., 1974).

acid for 10 to 15 hr, and analyzing the eluate by a polarographic method described previously (Vostal et al., 1974).

The study results are shown in Figure 2. Dust containing lead was found on the hands of inner city children and on inner city interior household surfaces in substantially larger amounts than in similar suburban settings. The fact that this lead could easily be rubbed off with a moist towel suggested that hand contamination might readily occur. Although adults reside in the same environment, they are less likely to wipe their hands on floors and sills, probably wash their hands more frequently, and certainly do not have the hand-to-mouth behavior characteristic of preschool children.

A clear relationship was evident between individual hand and household levels as well. Children with more than the median level of lead on their hands came predominantly from homes with a high lead content. All of the children with high hand levels (>30 μg/towel), were from homes with at least 90 μg of lead in the household specimens.

The study confirmed that lead contamination of the household dust in urban areas was not uncommon. We speculated as follows about the relative importance of pica for paint chips and contaminated hands as sources of lead.

1. Lead-containing peeling paint was found in about half the homes in the 1971 survey; although that is a disturbingly high figure, it also means that half the homes did not have an exposed source of lead paint. Pica affects a maximum of 20 to 30% of inner city children and is most common at 2 years of age (Barltrop, 1966). In other words, one child in eight might be expected both to have pica and to be in an environment with available leaded paint. With frequent household moving and day placement of children in other homes the exposure to peeling paint might be greater, but repeated swallowing of leaded paint would still appear to be the exception rather than the rule for the group of children studied.

2. The ubiquitous presence of lead in dust in these deteriorated homes could explain the observed change in the distribution curve of blood lead levels, with a slight upward shift of the mean value for the entire group rather than selected elevation of PbB values in a minority. Moreover, the persistence of elevated values until 5 yr of age is difficult to explain by pica alone, which usually

Table 1. Household dust lead.

Household Dust Values (μg/sample)	High PbB Group (N = 49)	Low PbB Group (N = 50)	P Values
Mean	265 (±288)	123(±160)	
Median	149	55	≤0.01
Combined group median (93 μg)			
Above median*	32	17	
Below median	17	33	0.005

*$\chi^2 = 9.7$.

disappears in all but a few children after 3 yr of age. Although intensive mouthing also diminishes after 2 or 3 years of age, dirty hands are more common, if anything, and hand-to-mouth activities do persist (Barltrop, 1966).

By the mid-1970's a number of observers had noted the presence of significant amounts of lead in household dust (Chisolm, 1973; Landrigan and Gelbach, 1975; Lepow et al., 1974; Needleman and Scanlon, 1973). Over the subsequent years several case reports suggested that lead dust brought into homes on the clothing of lead smelter workers is deposited on interior household surfaces to which children have access (Baker et al., 1977; Dolcourt et al., 1978; Gignere et al., 1977; Rice et al., 1977). These reports confirmed that the dirt-hand-mouth ingestion route was not only a theoretic possibility but a likely factor in these selected cases.

To explore further whether this mechanism of ingestion was significant for the majority of urban cases, we elected to compare children with high and low PbB living in the same inner city environment (Charney et al., 1980). Although a strong correlation between household dust lead and blood lead would not prove a causal link, failure to establish such a correlation would raise serious question about dust contamination as a meaningful factor. In addition, by studying multiple sources and mechanisms of lead exposure in the two groups, the relative importance of each factor (household dust, household paint and outside dirt lead) could be assessed.

Two groups of children from 18 to 72 mos of age were selected for study. The "high group" had at least two PbB determinations between 40 and 79 μg/dl and erythrocyte protoporphyrin (EP) values >59 μg/dl within a 4-mo period. The "low group" had PbB of <29 μg/dl and EP <59/dl in the 2 to 4 mos preceding the study. The groups were matched for sex, race and socioeconomic status. Children with PbB levels between 30 and 39 μg/dl were excluded from the sample to more sharply distinguish the two groups.

For study purposes, "home" was defined as all locations where the child had spent significant time in the prior four months. The following types of data were obtained through home visits:

1. Samples of outside soil, if the child was observed to play in the dirt,
2. samples of peeling paint or plaster in any area of the home,
3. samples of household dust and dirt on the hands of the child and all areas where he was said to play, collected by the alcohol towel wipe technique previously described (Sayre et al., 1974; Sayre and Katzel, 1979),
4. history of pica and mouthing activities including finger sucking and mouthing of toys or other objects and
5. amount of traffic on the street where the home was located.

The study results confirmed that household dust in the environment of children with elevated PbB levels contained significantly more lead than was found in the low PbB group (Table 1). In addition, more lead was found on the hands of

Table 2.   Hand lead level.

Hand Pb Level	High PbB Group (N = 49)	Low PbB Group (N = 50)	P Values
Mean	49 ± 69	21 ± 28	0.01
Median	30	12	
Combined group median (20 μg/sample)			
Above median*	31	16	
Below median	18	34	0.005

*$\chi^2 = 9.7$.

children with elevated PbB levels (Table 2). The two groups also differed significantly on a number of other variables (Table 3). There may be some question about the validity of the historic data on pica, however. All the high PbB children had already been so identified and questioned repeatedly by their own physicians about possible sources of lead exposure, particularly pica for paint. Although 22 of 49 parents of high PbB children reported pica for paint (compared to only 2 of 50 parents of low PbB families) only 7 of those 22 were in environments where the paint actually contained over 1% lead.

A number of individual factors were found to correlate with PbB, but no single correlation coefficient (R) exceeded 0.45. Therefore, no one variable explained more than 20% of the variance (R^2). To explore which combinations of factors might be important, a stepwise multiple regression analysis was performed. Table 4 lists the variables entered in order of significance for all age groups. The

Table 3.   Significant sources of lead and mechanism of ingestion.

	High PbB Group (N = 49)	Low PbB Group (N = 50)	P Values
*Mechanism of ingestion (by history)**			
Habitual finger sucking	73.5	50	0.04
Mouthing toys	82	58	0.007
Chewing pencils	50	24	0.001
Eating paint chips	43	4	0.001
Eating outside dirt	48	20	0.001
Source of lead			
Interior paint (% homes with ≥1% lead in paint)	46	26	0.05
Soil Pb†	(N = 36)	(N = 28)	
Mean value (μg/g)	1563 (±1325)	1008 (±899)	0.04
Median value (μg/g)	1502	633	

*Values are percent affected.
†Soil Pb values were compared by a student's t test, all other by χ^2 analysis.

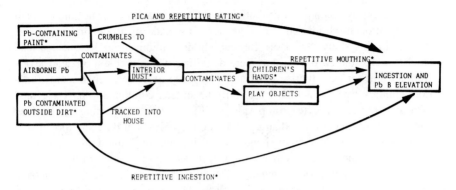

*SIGNIFICANT CORRELATION DEMONSTRATED IN PRESENT STUDY

Fig. 3. Possible mechanisms for blood Pb elevation of inner city children.

data were also analyzed by separate age groups (18 to 31, 33 to 47 and 48 to 72 mos). The analysis indicates that five or fewer factors greatly increase the amount of variance explained, from 44% for all children to 91% for black children 48 to 72 mos of age. Hand lead level, house dust lead level, lead in outside soil and a history of pica all appear to be multiplicative factors, contributing independently to the very high proportion of total variance explained. It is important to note that lead in interior paint did not prove a strong independent factor in any of the stepwise regression analyses.

In short, lead in interior dust and on the hands of children seemed to be a major factor in this study. The problem, however, is a multifactoral one with no single factor completely explaining the phenomenon. As indicated in Figure 3, a number of possible mechanisms and sources were found to be significant.

Table 4.   Stepwise multiple regression, all ages*.

Cumulative R^2 Values, Total Sample†		Cumulative R^2 Values Blacks Only‡	
0.21	Pica for paint	0.17	Soil Pb
0.33	Hand Pb	0.27	Household dust Pb
0.38	Eats outside dirt	0.34	Pica for paint
0.44	Household dust Pb	0.39	Finger sucking X hand Pb

*P < .0001. Values are entered in order of significance.
†For total sample, N = 99, R^2 = 0.44, F = 12.6.
‡For blacks only, N = 81, R^2 = 0.39, F = 10.3.

More recently, a major contribution to the understanding of the role of hand contamination in childhood lead ingestion was made by Roels and associates (1980). In this study, 11-yr-old Belgian children living in an area near a lead smelter were studied over a 4-yr period, during which ambient air lead levels from the smelter were markedly reduced. Despite this decrease in air contamination, children living less than 1 km from the smelter continued to have elevated PbB and free erythrocyte protoporphyrin (FEP) levels, suggesting a continued source of lead intake other than by inhalation. Analyses of dust and dirt in area playgrounds and of lead on the hands of the children (by a dilute nitric acid hand rinsing technique) clearly indicated that residual lead remained in the environment and did contaminate the hands of the children. Since 11-yr-olds do not have pica to any meaningful extent, and since the homes in the area did not contain lead-based paint, the implication is strong indeed that hand-to-mouth transfer of lead accounted for the increased body lead burden. Furthermore, PbB levels in boys were higher than those of girls living in the same area, and the hand levels of the boys were similarly higher, consistent with the observation of a greater degree of hand cleanliness in girls. The authors speculated that "hand contamination significantly influences blood lead concentration when lead . . . becomes higher than 20 μg/hand."

Although our studies in Rochester used a different method of hand lead analysis, we also observed that 20 μg/hand seems to be an important level. Only rarely did we find more than 20 μg on the hands of suburban children, urban children with normal PbB or adults.

What can we conclude about the role of hand contamination in the etiology of childhood lead ingestion? To summarize, a series of logical inferences can be made.

1. Lead has now been found in significant quantities in household and environmental dust and dirt where children are known to have elevated PbB levels. These observations have been made in Boston, New York City, Rochester, Hartford, El Paso, Northern Idaho, Baltimore, and cities in Belgium and Great Britain (Barltrop et al., 1975; Charney et al., 1980; Landrigan and Gehlbach, 1975; Lepow et al., 1974; Roels et al., 1980; Sayre et al., 1974; Yankel et al., 1977).

2. Within communities with high overall household dust lead levels, children have higher PbB than do adults from the same environment. (Landrigan and Gehlbach, 1975; Roels et al., 1980; Sayre et al., 1974).

3. The amount of lead on the hands of children correlates with lead both in the blood and in environmental dust and dirt (Charney et al., 1980; Roels et al., 1980).

4. Hand contamination with lead can be implicated as a factor in poisoning in cases where pica for paint or dirt, elevated ambient air levels or water contamination have been excluded (Baker et al., 1977; Dolcourt et al.,

1978; Gignere et al., 1977; Landrigan and Gehlbach, 1975; Rice et al., 1977; Roels et al., 1980).

It cannot be stated with certainty that for urban children in the United States hand contamination and mouthing of lead-containing household dust is the sole factor of sub-encephalopathic lead poisoning. On the contrary, evidence exists that a multiplicity of factors are involved. Moreover, a key piece of the puzzle remains to be elucidated, i.e., whether reduction of household dust levels can result in reduced blood lead levels. There is evidence that careful washing of windowsills and floor areas can reduce the dust lead levels markedly (Sayre and Katzel, 1972). These lead dust levels reaccumulate over a period of days to many weeks, depending on household traffic patterns, the general cleanliness of the house and whether or not windows are opened. At present a study is underway in Baltimore to assess whether specific types of periodic household cleaning can affect blood levels in children with moderate PbB elevation.

It does appear well established, however, that the role of household dust contamination needs to be considered if the problem of childhood lead poisoning is to be addressed. Even after ambient air levels are reduced in the instances of industrial pollution and after households with lead paint are scraped and repainted, the residue of contaminated dust and dirt in the environment remains a potent hazard for lead poisoning of children.

References

Baker, E., Folland, D., Taylor, T., Frank, M., Peterson, W., Lovejoy, Gr., Cox, D., Housworth, J, Landrigan, P. 1977. Lead poisoning in children of lead workers. Home contamination with industrial dust. NEJM 296:260.

Barltrop, D. 1966. The prevalence of pica. Am J Dis Child 112:116.

Barltrop, D., Strehlow, C., Thornton, I. and Webb, J. 1975. Absorption of lead from dust and soil. Postgrad Med J 51:801.

Charney, E., Sayre, J. and Coulter, M. 1980. Increased lead absorption in inner city children: Where does the lead come from? Pediat 65:226.

Chisolm, J. 1973. Screening for lead poisoning in children. Pediat 51:280.

Dolcourt, J., Hamrick, H., O'Tuama, L., Wooten, J., and Barker, E. L., 1978. Increased lead burden in children of battery workers: Asymptomatic exposure resulting from contaminated work clothing. Pediat 62:563.

Gignere, C., Howes, A., McBean, M. and Watson, W. 1977. Increased lead absorption in children of lead workers—Vermont. Morbid Mortal Weekly Rept 26:61.

Landrigan, P. and Gehlbach, S. 1975. Epidemic lead absorption near an ore smelter: The role of particulate lead. NEJM 292:123.

Lepow, M., Bruckman, L., Gillette, M., Markowitz, S., Robino, R., Kapish, J. 1974. Role of airborne lead in increased body burden of lead in Hartford children. Environ Health Perspect 7:99.

Morbid and Mortal Weekly Rept. 1980. 29:170.

Needleman, H. and Scanlon, J. 1973. Getting the lead out. NEJM 288:466.

Rice, C., Lilis, R., Fischbein, A. and Selikoff, I. 1977. Unsuspected sources of lead poisoning. NEJM 296:1416.

Roels, H., Bucket, J.P., Lauwerys, P., Bruaux, P., Claeys-Thoreau, F., Lafontaine, A., Verduyn, G. 1980. Exposure to lead by the oral and the pulmonary routes of children living in the vicinity of a primary lead smelter. Env Res 22:81.

Sayre, J.W, Charney, E., Vostal, J. and Pless, I.B. 1974. House and hand dust as a potential source of childhood lead exposure. Am J Dis Child 127:167.

Sayre, J. and Katzel, M. 1979. Household surface lead dust: Its accumulation in vacant homes. Environ Health Persp 29:179.

Vostal, J., Taves, E., Sayre, J.W. and Charney, E. 1974. Lead analysis of house dust: A method for detection of another source of lead exposure in inner city children. Environ Health Perspect 7:91.

Yankel, A., von Linden, I. and Walter, S. 1977. The Silver Valley lead study: The relationship between childhood blood lead levels and environmental exposure. J Air Poll Control Assn 27:763.

9. Social Factors in the Recurrence of Increased Lead Absorption in Children

David M. O'Hara

There is now so much lead in the environment that everyone is exposed to some extent. It is a major health hazard affecting both rural and urban children, although its effects are concentrated among the urban poor (Cohen et al., 1973). Residents of dilapidated inner city dwellings in which there has been an accumulation of dust from lead-based paint over many years constitute a large high risk group. Socioeconomic data from various studies clearly establish that children with lead poisoning primarily come from families with minimal income, few personal resources and poor nutritional habits (Oberle, 1969).

Until recently, undue lead absorption was thought to be primarily associated with pica behavior in young children (Lourie et al., 1963). It may still be the case that pica and its attendant large lead (Pb) intake has to be present for the development of clinical symptomatology. However, as Dr. Charney has pointed out (Chapter 8, more than 20 µg of lead on children's hands is associated with elevated blood lead levels. This is an infinitesimally small amount, easily picked up and ingested during the normal hand-to-mouth behavior of children, and certainly a far different problem for a mother to deal with than pica, which Dr. Cataldo discusses (Chapter 10). Perception of the problem is only slowly changing but it adds substantially to the burden faced by an already overwhelmed group. Effective management of children who have begun to show evidence of increasing blood levels of lead demands constant vigilance on the part of the homemaker over a period of years. Deteriorating houses painted with leaded paints constitute lead belts in many cities. These are heavily contaminated environments which only careful lead paint abatement and thorough ongoing house cleaning can combat.

As evidence continues to grow on the range of toxic effects of low levels of lead in humans (U.S. Environmental Protection Agency, 1977), strategies to deal with this problem have to be redefined. The extent of possible exposure, the nature of high risk groups, the combination of social and environmental factors influence the effectiveness of medical management, the costs of intervention at different levels of risk and the long-term costs of failure to intervene are just some of the issues to be considered in developing an appropriate public health program. These issues will be discussed in turn, with particular emphasis on one very high risk group of children, those experiencing repeated episodes of lead absorption. As used here, this high risk group consists of children who are re-exposed and whose blood lead level (PbB) rises above 50 μg/dl following each course of treatment. This, in turn, usually leads to one or more additional courses of chelation therapy.

Extent of Lead Toxicity in Children

Data reported from the Center for Disease Control (CDC) have shown remarkable consistency for the past several years. Approximately 7% of all children ages 1 to 5 yr screened for lead show evidence of lead toxicity as defined by the Center for Disease Control (1979b) (Table 1).

A positive screening test was defined in April, 1978, as an erythrocyte protoporphyrin (EP) $\geq$50 μg/dl of whole blood in association with a blood level $\geq$30 mg/dl.

The decline in the number of children screened per year has recently been reversed. This is primarily the result of expanded screening and reporting efforts by governmental programs providing services to children. These include the Early Periodic Screening, Diagnosis and Treatment Program (EPSDT) and the Maternal and Child Health Program of the Department of Health and Human Services, the well baby clinics in local health departments, and the U.S. Department of Agriculture, Special Supplemental Food Program for Women, Infants, and Children (WIC).

In fiscal year 1979 the number of children screened was at the highest level ever. Of the 464,751 children screened, 32,537 were found to have undue lead absorption. This is a substantial increase over the preceding year, with a gain of 16.8% in the number of children screened and 26.1% in the number of children found with undue lead absorption (Center for Disease Control, 1980).

Using the number of children reported with lead toxicity by these programs as the numerator and the entire U.S. population between 1 and 5 yrs of age as the denominator, the age-specific prevalence rate for calendar year 1978 was estimated as 175/100,000. The true prevalence rate is likely to be somewhat higher,

Table 1.   Lead poisoning. Number of children screened and found to have undue lead absorption in childhood lead-based paint poisoning prevention projects. United States, 1972-1978 (From MMWR 29:86).

Calendar Year	Estimated U.S. Population Ages 1-5	Number of Projects	Children				Identified with Iron Deficiency
			Screened		With Undue Lead Absorption		
			Number	Rate/ 100,000	Number	Rate/ 100,000	
1972	17,161,000	37	119,960	699	9,044	53	NA
1973	16,999,000	42	296,879	1,746	19,059	112	NA
1974	16,690,000	77	449,318	2,692	24,443	146	NA
1975	16,294,000	77	421,338	2,586	30,343	186	4,062
1976	15,831,000	66	406,413	2,559	33,043	208	10,103
1977	15,339,000	65	381,201	2,485	28,072	183	15,896
1978	15,236,000	64	410,211	2,692	26,734	175	17,069
Total			2,485,320		170,738		47,130

but accurate estimates are difficult to establish. Even with this figure, the age-specific attack rate exceeds the rates reported for most childhood diseases (Center for Disease Control, 1979a).

Current screening programs are aimed primarily at children under 6 yrs old who live in deteriorating inner city areas. Estimates place the number of such highly exposed children at 1.5 million and the total number of children under 6 yrs at 15 million. Thus, current screening programs examine less than 30% of the targeted high risk group and less than 3% of all children under 6 yrs. Available prevalence data indicate that screening efforts should continue to expand since the point of diminishing returns, which is a smaller proportion of children identified as at risk, has not yet been reached.

High Risk Groups

Aggregate prevalence figures conceal the especially important issue of the extent of exposure experienced by different groups. This can be viewed in two ways, the number of screened children falling into the higher CDC risk categories III and IV and the number of children found to have moved into a higher CDC risk category upon follow-up (see Table 1, Chapter 1, for CDC risk classification). For the second quarter of fiscal year 1979, 29.8% of the children found to have undue lead absorption were in CDC risk categories III and IV, an increase of 15.1% over the same period in fiscal year 1978 (Center for Disease Control, 1979c). This trend toward an increase in the proportion of children identified in screening risk classifications III and IV continued through the remainder of fiscal year 1979 (Center for Disease Control, 1980). It is a disturbing trend after almost a decade of effort to screen and treat children with lead toxicity.

The second group of children who cause concern is composed of those whose risk classification status increases between reporting periods. The children in this category suffer chronic exposure and constitute a small but fairly constant proportion of the total number of children screened. In the second quarter of 1979, 17,602 children were reported to be under pediatric management for lead toxicity. Of these, 18.3% (3,216) were reported to be at reduced risk. However, 3.2% (557) of the children who were re-evaluated had increased risk. During the third quarter of fiscal year 1979, the percentage at increased risk remained unchanged (Center for Disease Control, 1979d). Although this number is small, it causes concern because an increase in risk normally reflects failure to identify and eliminate the hazardous source of lead in the child's environment. Prolonged exposure also increases the length of treatment, the likelihood of permanent sequellae and the stress experienced by the families of these children (Albert et al., 1974; Pueschel et al., 1972; Rummo, 1977). The available figures may also be a significant underestimation of the extent of chronic exposure. In a report prepared for the Center for Disease Control evaluating the effectiveness of selected childhood screening programs, it was found that between 20 and 25% of the cases studied failed to improve (Kennedy, 1978).

The importance of shortening the period of exposure was confirmed by data presented by Rummo (1977). Children exposed to lead levels of 40 μg/dl for less than 6 mos were no different from controls on measures of cognitive performance. Exposure over 6 mos was associated with poorer performance. Albert et al. (1974) and Pueschel et al. (1972) also have data which suggest that therapeutic intervention reduces injury.

For the remainder of this paper, attention will be focused on the group of children who either experience an increase in risk status over time or experience repeated episodes of significantly increased lead absorption.

Social Risk Factors

Relatively few studies have focused on the social risk factors associated with chronic childhood lead poisoning. The possible combination of social, familial and environmental factors involved has been subject to clinical assessment but little systematic review. Early studies emphasized the interactions of lead-based paint and persistent pica in the development of lead poisoning (Layman et al., 1963; Lourie, 1971; Lourie et al., 1963; Millican et al., 1956). Causal factors proposed were childrearing practices and cultural patterns which supported pica behavior (Barltrop, 1959). One longitudinal study of children with pica has been done (Bicknell, 1975). In this study, there was the serendipitous occurrence of natural controls, siblings of the children with pica who also developed lead poisoning during the course of the study. For both groups of children, the same combination of circumstances existed: families living in a state of deprivation, subject to social disorganization and poverty, with a lack of parental supervision, and the ready availability of crumbling lead paint in substandard housing. Pica behavior alone was not sufficient to identify children with lead poisoning.

Other studies have confirmed the association between socioeconomic status of families and several risk-related variables, such as residence, family life style and access to medical information (Albert et al., 1974; Barltrop, 1969; Cohen et al., 1973; Hale and Lepow, 1971; Hunter, 1977; Lepow et al., 1974; Margulis, 1977; Meigs and Whitmore, 1971; Peuschel et al., 1972; Stark et al., 1978). Characteristics of adults in families also may contribute to a child's exposure to lead. For example, marital status, poor supervision, number of adults in the household, number and ages of children, cultural and individual variations in parent-child interactions and differences in household cleaning practices all may affect exposure to lead (Barltrop, 1969; Chisolm and Kaplan, 1968).

Two studies have sought specifically to contribute to an understanding of the familial contribution to the likelihood of chronic lead poisoning. The first describes a project aimed at comparing the familial characteristics of children hospitalized with lead poisoning with those of children hospitalized with two other conditions, inguinal hernia and pneumonia (Meigs and Whitmore, 1971). Families with lead-poisoned children were more likely to be black, have a marital separation, have a father unemployed, have a mother employed or at school, have a greater number of children in the family, have the hospitalized child be supervised by someone other than the mother, live in poor housing and receive public assistance.

This study subsequently was extended to cover approximately 90% of children ages 1 to 6 yrs living in New Haven, Connecticut (Stark et al., 1978). Results confirmed the nature of the familial variables associated both with the initial risk of the child having an elevated blood lead level and the likelihood of a recurrence of excessive lead absorption. The Connecticut data suggest a relationship between four primary familial characteristics and an elevated blood lead level in the child. These characteristics were: number of children under 6 years in the home, number of parents in the home, employment status of parents and day care for the child. They suggest an association between family management, particularly an index of parental supervision or an adequate substitute (day care) and the risk of developing lead poisoning.

In a much smaller study by Chaiklin et al. (1974), a pattern of continued exposure was found to be associated with two maternal characteristics, level of education and employment status. The lead-poisoned groups were differentiated in terms of a single treated episode versus repeated elevated blood lead levels. In the repeated episode families, it was found that there was a greater proportion of marital difficulties, problems in adult adjustment and poor child rearing practices. However, these were differences only of degree; both groups were in a struggle for survival. According to Chaiklin et al. (1974), "they suffer from a lack of income, poor housing, unemployment and under-employment."

The significance of these studies is that they go beyond the general high risk status of poor urban children and begin to address the characteristics of the group at highest risk. To some extent, the findings may be self-evident, but for treatment purposes they confirm the social as well as environmental nature of chronic lead poisoning.

Environmental Risk

Among the many sources of environmental exposure to lead, housing has long held the most critical position despite recent attention to the potential role of airborne lead from automobile exhausts (Lepow et al., 1974; U.S. Environmental Protection Agency, 1977). Ongoing follow-up of children treated by the Lead Poisoning Program at the John F. Kennedy Institute has provided some preliminary data which indicate a very strong link between housing conditions and recurrence of lead toxicity.

The Clinic primarily draws its patients from the lower socioeconomic groups. The housing available falls into four general types, classified according to the degree of environmental lead exposure in and around the home:

Type A. Low Lead Exposure

1. Modern housing (less than approximately 15 yrs old located on periphery of city).
2. Public housing projects ("lead free"), with many located in the inner city.

Type B. Modestly Increased Lead Exposure

1. Totally renovated inner city housing.
2. Old housing completely abated relative to lead hazards.

Type C. Moderately Increased Lead Exposure

Old inner city housing abated (partial, i.e., up to 4-ft level) for lead hazard, according to local ordinances.

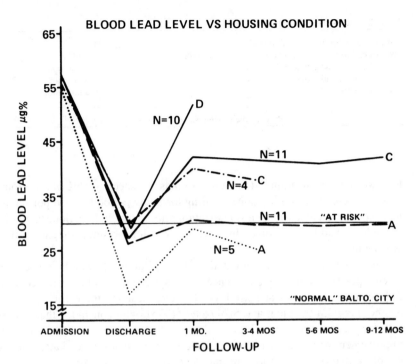

Fig. 1. Blood lead levels over time *versus* degree of environmental lead exposure of child's dwelling. A, low lead exposure; C, moderately increased lead exposure; D, high lead exposure. Subjects A and C had only been followed for 3-4 mos.

Type D. High Lead Exposure

Old inner city housing containing lead pigment paints flaking and chipping from various interior and exterior surfaces.

In a preliminary study children were followed for up to 1 yr subsequent to an initial hospitalization. The general practice was to hospitalize preschool-aged children with confirmed PbB in excess of 50 μg Pb/dl whole blood. Discharge from hospital was keyed primarily to the location for a family of housing with significantly reduced environmental lead exposure. Figure 1 shows the pattern of blood lead level change over time in terms of the type of housing to which the child returned. Only the children discharged to lead-free public housing remain below the accepted CDC risk cut-off point of 30 μg Pb/dl. The ten children discharged to Type D housing with continued high lead exposure all experienced a return to the 50 μg/dl hospitalization criterion within 1 month following discharge.

The Kennedy Institute Lead Clinic mainly refers children to two hospitals in Baltimore for inpatient treatment. Over a 1-yr period, 34 different children with

Table 2.   Excess hospitalization.

No. of Pb children admitted in study year	34
No. of children with repeat admission (any hospital)	19 (56%)
No. of children admitted × 2 = 13	26 admissions
No. of children admitted × 3 = 4	12 admissions
No. of children admitted × 4 = 2	8 admissions
19	46
Preventable readmissions =	27

lead poisoning were admitted to these hospitals. Nineteen or 56% of this group of children were either rehospitalized during the study period for lead poisoning or had experienced at least one hospitalization prior to the study period. In all, these 19 children had been involved in 46 admissions for the single diagnosis of lead poisoning.

This is not necessarily representative of all children followed by this clinic. It refers specifically to the experience of hospitalized children who continued follow-up treatment for at least 1 yr. The data bear out the earlier analysis of another program by Klein and Schlageter (1975), who concluded that intensive follow-up combined with effective abatement of sources resulted in a marked improvement of blood lead levels in children, but when source abatement could not be carried out, other forms of intervention were ineffective.

Treatment Costs

It is possible to derive estimates of the excess treatment costs incurred by this group of children. Using the average length of stay (15 days) for children admitted with the primary diagnosis of lead poisoning and the average daily hospitalization cost ($350), the excess hospitalization cost for nineteen children is over $140,000.

Abatement Costs

In 1979, estimates of the cost of abatement of the typical family dwelling in Philadelphia ranged from $900 to $1500 (W. Sobolesky, personal communication). Earlier figures on housing abatement costs from the Department of Housing and Urban Development provide a national perspective (Billick and Gray, 1978).

Table 3.   Estimated hospitalization costs.

Excess hospitalization cost for repeat admission	$ 141,750
Average cost of one hospitalization	$ 5,250
Total hospitalization cost of all Pb admissions	$ 241,500

Using the Philadelphia figures for the cost of abatement, there are substantial treatment versus abatement cost comparisons for the group of recurrent exposure children treated by the John F. Kennedy Institute Lead Poisoning Program. Hospitalization costs total $141,750 compared with an estimated $28,500 for housing abatement. Follow-up clinic visits at $40 per visit might add to these figures a $160 treatment cost per child in the first year, or a total of $3,040 for 19 children. If follow-up continued for a further 3 yr, with two clinic visits per year, this would generate an additional $4,560 in treatment costs. But these costs would remain necessary with or without housing abatement because of the pervasive nature of urban lead exposure. Potential net savings if housing abatement was successful in leading to the prevention of repeat hospitalization remain in excess of $100,000 for these 19 children. Providing the additional social services associated with the prevention of chronic lead toxicity, such as day care, homemaker services, social work support, nutrition, education and pediatric nurse practitioner services can still be accomplished with such substantial cost savings.

Similar estimates are not readily available for the cost of outpatient treatment and follow-up. At a minimum, they would have to include an initial course of 5 days of outpatient chelation therapy following the screening and diagnostic visits. The follow-up period should extend through at least the high risk period of a child's life with subsequent screening at 1- to 3-mo intervals, according to the Center for Disease Control. The Center for Disease Control guidelines recommend that all children 1 to 6 yr old should be followed continuously if they live in or frequently visit poorly maintained homes built prior to the 1960's, or if they may be exposed to other more specific hazardous lead sources such as lead smelters (U.S. Department of Health, Education and Welfare, 1979). Long term follow-up is not an inexpensive proposition and may have to include several

Table 4.   1977 estimates of the cost of lead paint removal.

1. From pre1940 dwellings with lead content in paint 2.0 milligram/square centimeter	Cost per dwelling unit: $1,070
2. All dwellings containing lead-based paint with	National costs:
a) 5 milligrams/square centimeter	$20 billion
b) 1.5 milligrams/square centimeter	$55 billion
3. To remove only peeling and flaking paint on pre1940 dwellings	Cost per unit: $215 National: $2.1 billion

children in some families. The cost comparisons with housing abatement deserve further study if effective treatment is to be the goal.

The figures presented above represent only clearly identifiable costs. Failure to prevent chronic exposure to lead is known to be accompanied by permanent neurological sequellae which may lead to additional special education costs, in severe cases to the costs of residential care, and reduced earnings potential in adulthood (Chisolm, 1970; Conley, 1973).

Policy Implications

The cost estimates and recurrence data presented here refer only to the experience of Baltimore City. They are suggestive but not conclusive. For program and policy development, further research is needed to compare equivalent costs for appropriate follow up and retreatment of children who continue to be exposed (Klein and Schlageter, 1975; Pueschel et al., 1972). Thus far, this is an unexamined issue. However, the experience of children with recurrent lead toxicity parallels what is known about other major contributors to health costs. Repeat hospitalization for the same disease is a substantial factor in driving up health expenditures. Typically, the high cost patients are not those in intensive care nor in a terminal condition. They constitute a group for whom medical advances have reduced mortality rates while increasing the average duration of the illness and the need for multiple hospitalizations (Greenberg, 1977).

Children suffering from lead toxicity fall into a different category. If long term neurological sequellae of low levels of exposure are confirmed, the resulting costs are likely to fall on educational programs in the form of special educational provision to deal with learning and behavioral difficulties. In the short term, treatment can reduce the body lead burden substantially and at least medically cure the acute problem. The cost burden then shifts and is much more difficult to establish.

Thus far, health policy has largely ignored the issue of chronicity among children with lead poisoning. This neglect not only constitutes a real problem in designing and funding appropriate treatment programs for lead poisoned children, but also ignores the substantial preventable costs incurred.

Enough is now known about the problem of lead toxicity in children to make medical treatment a reliable and predictable intervention. Body levels of lead in young children who have not suffered chronic exposure can be brought down to relatively safe levels fairly quickly and the attendant risk for any permanent neurological damage minimized. The prevention of repeated exposure to sources of lead in the environment is critical to effective long term management. To be successful, this aspect of treatment leaves the immediate medical arena and demands priorities in social and health care policy which can be responsive to environmental and familial problems (Chaiklin, 1979). Without effective programs of housing abatement or rehousing and supportive services to families often faced with significant additional emotional and financial costs in providing appropriate care, the experience of one group of children in Baltimore is likely to be repeated.

Efforts to develop a clear national health policy on the treatment of lead toxicity in children reflect current realities (U.S. Department of Health, Education and Welfare, 1978). Belief that the source of exposure for children is primarily pica behavior and the ingestion of lead paint chips is only gradually changing. Appreciation of the importance of leaded dust which has accumulated over time and is conveyed to the mouth during normal play activity is just beginning to grow. (See Chapter 8.)

This change in understanding suggests a change in the recommended standard for housing abatement away from the removal of all lead-based paint to the strict control of flaking and peeling paint and through clean-up procedures which can reduce and control the leaded dust level in the house. The economic analysis of different standards for abatement already exists. In the past, the prohibitively expensive cost estimates of a national lead paint abatement program based on total lead paint removal acted as an effective barrier to a broad national program of intervention. Focusing on flaking and peeling paint as the hazard and dust control as a potentially significant preventive activity should permit the reassessment of priorities, especially as more evidence emerges of the gradually accumulating economic costs of the failure to take preventive measures.

The implication of repeat hospitalization for health policy also involves the design of health insurance, particularly the Medicaid program, since it currently is the major source of reimbursement for the excess hospitalization of children with lead toxicity. Currently, there are no financial incentives in the Medicaid program for efforts to prevent repeat hospitalization. One option might be to include in the Medicaid program reimbursement of the costs of environmental inspection and abatement for the high risk group. Another option is to require, as part of the Medicaid reimbursement plan, that provision be made for adequate enforcement of abatement measures and supportive social services if health care dollars are to be spent.

So far, Federal policies and programs to deal with this issue of lead poisoning have reflected the substantial economic forces at play. Because it brings together a broad array of special interests involved with housing, environment and health issues, the gradually evolving understanding of the nature, extent and impact of the problem has fueled an ongoing debate.

Whereas it was once seen as a critical problem only for the urban poor, there is now a wider arena of concern. This is at once an asset and a liability. The costs of a broadly based strategy to eliminate the problem are overwhelming. Politically, to acquiesce in the status quo is the most favored path. These cost and political considerations combine to make efforts to target effective services on the group at highest risk difficult to implement. It seems clear that broadly based screening efforts should continue to expand. They have been shown to be effective at significantly reducing encephalopathy and death, as well as in identifying children with lead toxicity prior to the onset of clinical symptoms. The identified iron-deficient group also benefits substantially from improved nutritional programs.

Risk containment and the prevention of recurrence is a more complex issue. It seems that there is an as yet unexplored middle ground between the complete elimination of exposure to lead as a goal and the programs designed to use all effective preventive measures with high risk groups. If the Baltimore experience is repeated elsewhere, not necessarily in terms of repeat hospitalization, but perhaps through successive episodes of outpatient treatment, then health care costs multiply rapidly. The cost data presented above tend to support a health care strategy for a group of children at high risk for repeated exposure which includes housing abatement, dust control and social support to families as an integral part of treatment in order to prevent the unnecessary costs of recurrent exposure.

References

Albert, R.E., Shore, R.E., Sayers, A.J., Strehlow, C., Kneip, T.J., Pasternack, B.S., Friedhoff, A.J., Covan, F. and Cimino, J.A. 1974. Follow-up of children overexposed to lead. Environ Health Perspec 7:33–40.

Barltrop, D. 1959. Aetiology of pica. Lancet 2:515.

Barltrop, D. 1969. Factors influencing exposure of children to lead. Arch Dis Childh 44:476.

Bicknell, J. 1975. Pica: A childhood symptom. Butterworth and Company, London.

Billick, I.H. and Gray, V.E. 1978. Lead based paint poisoning research: Review and evaluation 1971–1977. Office of Policy Development and Research. U.S. Department of Housing and Urban Development, Washington.

Center for Disease Control, 1979a. Morbidity and Mortality Weekly Reports, March 16, 1979.

Center for Disease Control. 1979b. Morbidity and Mortality Weekly Reports. September 14, 1979.

Center for Disease Control. 1979c. Morbidity and Mortality Weekly Reports. September 21, 1979.

Center for Disease Control. 1979d. Morbidity and Mortality Weekly Reports, October 19, 1979.

Center for Disease Control. 1980. Morbidity and Mortality Weekly Reports. April 18, 1980.

Chaiklin, H. 1979. The treadmill of lead. Orthopsychiatry 49:571–573.

Chaiklin, H., Cook, J.J., Hayes, M.E. and Scanland, V.B. 1974. Recurrence of lead poisoning in children. Social Work 19:196–200.

Chisolm, J.J., Jr. 1970. Lead poisoning in children and its prevention. In: Hearings on S. 3216, pp. 206–215. U.S. Senate Committee in Labor and Public Welfare, Subcommittee on Health, 91st Congress, 2nd Session, Washington.

Chisolm, J.J., Jr. and Kaplan, E. 1968. Lead poisoning in childhood—comprehensive management and prevention. J Pediat 73:942–950.

Cohen, C.J., Bowers, G.N. and Lepow, M.L. 1973. Epidemiology of lead poisoning: A comparison between urban and rural children. JAMA 226:1430–1433.

Conley, R.W. 1973. The economics of mental retardation. Johns Hopkins University Press, Baltimore.

Greenberg, E.M. 1977. The failure of success. Millbank Mem Fund Q 55:3–24.

Hale, M. and Lepow, M.L. 1971. Epidemiology of increased lead exposure among 954 one–five year old Hartford, Connecticut children—1970. Conn Med 35:492–497.

Hunter, J.M. 1977. The summer disease—an integrative model of the seasonality aspects of childhood lead poisoning. Soc Sci Med 11:691–703.

Kennedy, F.D. 1978. The childhood lead poisoning prevention program: An evaluation. Environmental Health Services Division, Center for Disease Control, U.S. Public Health Service, Atlanta (Unpublished manuscript).

Klein, M.C. and Schlageter, M. 1975. Nontreatment of screened children with intermediate blood lead levels. Ped 56:298–302.

Layman, E.M., Millican, F.K., Lourie, R.S. and Takahashi, L.Y. 1963. Cultural influences and symptom choice: Clay eating customs in relation to the etiology of pica. Psychol Rec 13:249.

Lepow, M.L., Bruckman, L., Rubino, R.A., Markowtiz, S., Gillette, M. and Kapish, J. 1974. Role of airborne lead in increased body burden of lead in Hartford children. Environ Health Perspec 7:99–102.

Lourie, R. 1971. Prevention of lead paint—or prevention of pica? Ped 48:490–491.

Lourie, R.S., Layman, E.M. and Millican, F.K. 1963. Why children eat things that are not food. Children 10:144.

Margulis, H.L. 1977. The control and prevention of pediatric lead poisoning in East Orange, New Jersey. Environ Health 39:362–365.

Meigs, J.W. and Whitmore, E. 1971. Epidemiology of lead poisoning in New Haven children: Operational factors. Conn Med 35:363–369.

Milican, F.K., Lourie, R.S. and Layman, E.M. 1956. Emotional factors in the etiology and treatment of lead poisoning. Am J Dis Child 91:144–149.

Oberle, M.W. 1969. Lead poisoning: A preventable childhood disease of the slums. Science 165:991–992.

Pueschel, S.M., Kopito, L. and Schwachman, H. 1972. Children with an increased lead burden: A screening and follow-up study. JAMA 222:462.

Rummo, J.H. 1974. Intellectual and behavioral effects of lead poisoning in children. Ph.D. thesis, University of North Carolina, Chapel Hill, N.C., Ann Arbor, Mich., University of Mich., Microfilms, as cited in 1977 EPA-600/8-77-017, Chapter 11, pp 11-21.

Stark, A.D., Meigs, J.W., Fitch, R.A. and DeLouise, E.R. 1978. Family operational cofactors in the epidemiology of childhood lead poisoning. Arch Environ Health Sept-Oct:222–225.

U.S. Department of Health, Education, and Welfare. Center for Disease Control. 1978. Preventing lead poisoning in young children. A statement by the Center for Disease Control, Atlanta, DHEW, PHS, CDC (00-2629).

U.S. Department of Health, Education, and Welfare. Bureau of Community Health Services and Center for Disease Control. 1979. Joint statement: Lead poisoning in children, Washington.

U.S. Environmental Protection Agency. Office of Research and Development. 1977. Air quality criteria for lead. Washington. EPA-600/8-77-017.

10. Behavioral Approaches to Lead Ingestion

Michael F. Cataldo, Jack W. Finney,
Nancy A. Madden, and Dennis C. Russo

Introduction

Lead poisoning of children is a problem with a variety of solutions. One major method by which children absorb lead is through the ingestion of lead-based paint either in the form of paint chips or finer paint particles which are present in many older, poorly maintained houses. Lead paint chips may be directly ingested (pica). Dust containing lead may also be ingested during hand-to-mouth behavior when the child puts toys or body parts exposed to the dust into his mouth (Sayre et al., 1974). Sachs et al. (1970) found that 78% of children with moderate to severe lead poisoning exhibited pica, and Lin Fu (1973) estimated that 60 to 80% of severe lead poisoning cases occur as a result of pica.

Since lead ingestion occurs primarily because of pica and mouthing, a possible solution is the use of behavior modification techniques to reduce the occurrence of these behaviors. Pica and mouthing related to items other than lead paint have been successfully modified in profoundly retarded institutionalized individuals, through the use of behavioral procedures including brief restraint (Bucher et al., 1976), time-out from interaction and activities (Ausman et al., 1974) and oral hygiene over-correction procedures (Foxx and Azrin, 1973; Foxx and Martin, 1975). Unfortunately, few parallels exist between institutionalized retarded pop-

The research reported here and the preparation of this paper was supported in part by Grant No. 917 from the Maternal and Child Health Services and is part of a collaborative effort of the John F. Kennedy Institute and the Behavioral Medicine Program of The Johns Hopkins University School of Medicine.

ulations and young children exposed to lead paint hazards. As opposed to the punishment procedures used with institutionalized populations, less restrictive educational techniques can reduce pica in the child at risk for lead poisoning. For example, Baer (1962) and Lowitz and Suib (1978) have found that reinforcing a child when he was not engaged in thumbsucking, a procedure referred to as differential reinforcement of other behavior (DRO), was effective in modifying this behavior, which is present in many children with pica. In young children for whom developmental and learning considerations play a prominent role, other approaches based on stimulus control (teaching children what materials are not to be put in the mouth) or skill development (teaching them ways of playing that do not involve mouthing) might be equally successful in reducing pica while providing a less restrictive treatment approach. This may be especially appropriate, given the often permissive cultural attitudes toward pica (Chatterjee and Gettman, 1972) and the accompanying lack of education about pica (de la Burde and Reames, 1973) which characterize the population at risk.

Behavioral studies on pica in children at risk for lead poisoning are noticeably absent in both the behavioral and lead poisoning literatures. For this reason a series of analogue studies have been initiated at the John F. Kennedy Institute to determine some relevant variables and the effectiveness of behavioral procedures as a solution to the problem of lead poisoning. The first study is described in Figure 1 showing that mouthing of both objects and body parts occurs more in an impoverished setting than in a setting enriched with play materials or with a number of other children and adults present (Madden et al., 1980a).

Behavioral Approaches for Reducing Pica and Mouthing

The purpose of the analogue studies was to determine the effectiveness of behavioral procedures in reducing pica and mouthing behavior under somewhat ideal conditions. The basic procedures were as follows. Children hospitalized for treatment of asymptomatic lead intoxication were observed in a variety of hospital situations. In one situation, a room with a one-way mirror and microphone/speaker system was equipped with a variety of household items and a Masonite board coated with a flour and water paste mix which, after drying, resembled flaking paint. Some chips from this dried mix were spread on a nearby table, on the windowsill and on the floor near the board. These simulated chips resembled chips of real paint quite closely; when subjects were asked to identify the simulated paint chips, they said ''paint'' without hesitation.

Three intervention procedures were employed in a multiple baseline design, with more restrictive and intensive procedures used only if those less so proved

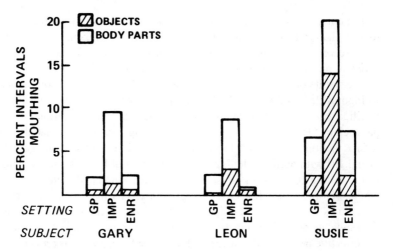

Fig. 1. Mean percentages of intervals in which mouthing of objects, mouthing of body parts and total mouthing were observed across sessions for each subject in three settings, group play environment (GP), impoverished individual play environment (IMP), and enriched individual play environment (ENR). Total mouthing is represented by combining the percentage intervals for mouthing body parts and mouthing of objects. Reprinted with permission from Journal of Pediatric Psychology 5:207–216.

ineffective. The first procedure was discrimination training, in which children immediately prior to each session were reinforced for correctly stating whether particular items presented to them were edible or not. This procedure would eliminate pica if a child was ignorant of the inappropriateness of mouthing or eating particular items. The next procedure employed was correspondence training, in which the child was rewarded for accurately reporting on his or her pica behavior in the experimental setting. For very young children who did not have good language skills and therefore could not report on their behavior, rewards were provided when the child engaged in behavior other than pica. This procedure is referred to as differential reinforcement of other behavior (DRO). During this intervention, children were reinforced for the absence of pica based on direct observation. The last intervention was an overcorrection procedure designed to punish pica because it was a potentially dangerous activity. The overcorrection procedure consisted of brushing the mouth and teeth of the child for 1 min with a soft bristle toothbrush dipped in Listerine mouthwash every time pica occurred. The overcorrection was always used with the DRO procedure, so that if a child did not engage in pica there was always a positive consequence. While even a mild punitive procedure clearly is not a preferred method in changing the behavior of young children, it was felt that the danger the behavior carried for children warranted its use.

The criterion for success for any particular intervention was a reduction of pica to less than 3% of the intervals observed. This stringent criterion was used because very small amounts of lead can produce toxic effects, so that even low levels of pica are dangerous.

The results of the first intervention study (Madden et al., 1980b) are presented in Figures 2, 3 and 4. For the first subject, a 5.5-yr-old girl, with low average intelligence, the discrimination training procedure successfully reduced pica of paint chips. However, correspondence training had to be initiated in order to reduce mouthing of objects to the criterion level. The second subject was a 2.5-yr-old girl with normal intelligence. Observation of her behavior was made both in the testing room (with household items and simulated paint chips) and in a similar setting in which a variety of play materials were available. Intervention procedures were employed only in the testing room (Impoverished Setting). The data indicate that discrimination and correspondence training procedures were not effective but that DRO successfully reduced pica, and this reduction general-

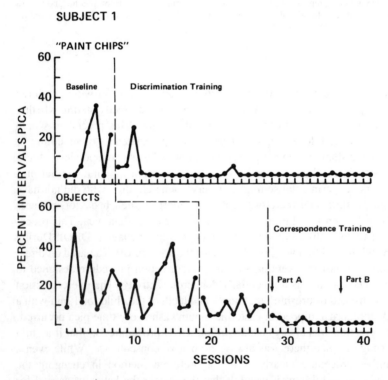

Fig. 2. Occurrence of pica of "paint chips" and objects during the phases of treatment for Subject 1. Reprinted with permission from *Child Behavior Therapy* 2:67–81.

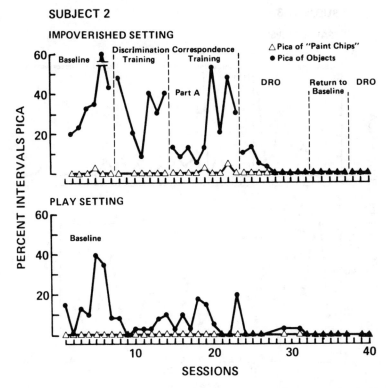

Fig. 3. Occurrence of pica of ''paint chips'' and objects in two settings for Subject 2. Reprinted with permission from *Child Behavior Therapy* 2:67–81.

ized from the Impoverished to the Play Setting. For the third subject, a 2-yr-old girl of normal intelligence, discrimination training and the DRO procedure reduced pica below baseline levels, but only the DRO plus overcorrection reduced and maintained pica below the criterion for success.

Although clearly not exhaustive in its examination of all treatment possibilities or combinations, this pilot intervention study did suggest that pica behavior of children with lead poisoning could be reduced by behavioral procedures. Accordingly, a second demonstration study was conducted (Finney et al., in press) in which four children also hospitalized for treatment of asymptomatic lead intoxication were provided with the same behavioral treatment package of discrimination training, DRO, and DRO plus overcorrection. The setting and procedures were the same as those described in the first intervention study. The results are shown in Figure 5. The subjects as presented in Figure 5 were a boy, 3 yr 6 mos, with an IQ of 55 (John), a boy, 3 yr 9 mos, with an IQ of 75 (Sam), a girl, 5 yr 8 mos, with an IQ of 68 (Pam) and a girl, 2 yr 3 mos, with an IQ of 112

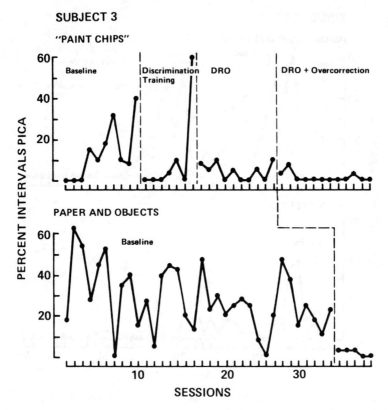

Fig. 4. Occurrence of pica of "paint chips" and objects during the phases of treatment for Subject 3. Reprinted with permission from *Child Behavior Therapy* 2:67–81.

(Nancy). The results demonstrate that the treatment package was effective in reducing the pica behavior of each child in the controlled hospital setting. The discrimination training and DRO procedures were effective for two children; the overcorrection procedure was necessary to maintain low amounts of pica in the other two children. It is also noteworthy that even though mouthing was greatly reduced in these two studies, the children continued to contact and to play with materials at pre-intervention levels. This pilot study was conducted in the hospital; the potential utility of this approach in outpatient settings remains to be evaluated.

The success of behavioral procedures depends on the degree to which they are carried out. Even under the best conditions, more positive and less punishing behavioral procedures will likely reduce but not eliminate pica and mouthing. The appropriateness of behavioral procedures as a solution to the problem of lead ingestion is determined by the level of pica (and thus lead ingestion) that is considered acceptable. Since some amounts of lead can be found in commonly available foodstuffs, no additional intake of lead should be acceptable. If no less than total reduction is acceptable, then behavioral procedures do not represent a satisfactory solution and will provide little or no benefit. In fact, if use of behavioral procedures prevents the employment of other solutions to the lead ingestion problem, then behavioral procedures not only are of no benefit, but represent a real risk. In light of the probable results from a behavior modification program to prevent lead ingestion and the lack of research on such programs in the literature, it would be incorrect to conclude at this time that such programs would provide an acceptable single solution. In particular, one should not conclude that programs to de-lead housing be abandoned in favor of programs which change the mouthing and pica behavior of children. If the ultimate goal is to insure that children do not ingest lead paint chips or dust, and behavioral procedures cannot guarantee this, then removal of lead paint from the environment is the most rational and imperative course of action. A case in point is the

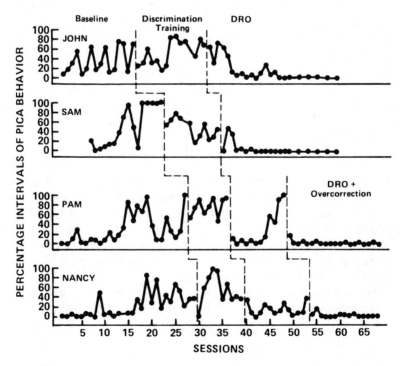

Fig. 5. Percentage of intervals in which pica behavior was observed across experimental conditions for the four subjects. Reprinted with permission from *Journal of Pediatric Psychology*. In press.

fact that for the four children in the last intervention analogue study, follow-up data strongly suggest that blood lead concentrations decreased in relation to a change in overall exposure of the child.

However, if other methods for reducing lead absorption are not withheld, then we probably should proceed with developing behavior modification approaches, inasmuch as they reduce the risk of lead ingestion but in themselves provide no appreciable inherent risks. Indeed, behavior modification may offer substantial benefit in selected cases, such as those of severe pica, in which are found very high blood lead levels and the attendent risk of symptomatic plumbism.

The most effective use of a behavioral program to reduce pica of children at high risk for lead poisoning would be as a preventative measure provided on an outpatient basis. The success of such a program is largely dependent upon parental compliance with the procedures recommended. While parents often do not comply with health-related suggestions, the seriousness of the consequences of lead poisoning to the developing child presents an important incentive. In addition, frequent clinic and public health nurse visits can greatly improve parental compliance with the program.

Another factor influencing program success is the frequency of pica behavior. Since learning takes place as a function of the consequences which occur for particular behaviors, the more frequently a behavior occurs the more rapidly appropriate learning can be programmed. Unfortunately, serious lead poisoning can occur with as few as one or two ingestions of paint residue per week, a behavioral rate that requires a long time for learning to take place.

Conclusion

The serious problem of lead poisoning of children has been related to lead-based paint, particularly in older housing. One method for lead absorption is believed to be the hand-to-mouth behavior which is engaged in by all children during normal development. Recent analogue research has shown that in a small number of children hospitalized with high lead levels, pica and mouthing were inversely related to the availability of environmental stimuli and could be modified by reinforcement and punishment techniques.

The utility of behavior procedures to reduce hand-to-mouth behavior (and thus lead poisoning) in home settings has not yet been demonstrated.

References

Ausman, J., Ball, T.S. and Alexander, D. 1974. Behavior therapy of pica in a profoundly retarded adolescent. Mental Retardation 12:16–18.

Baer, D.M. 1962. Laboratory control of thumbsucking in three young children by withdrawal and re-presentation of positive reinforcement. Journal Experimental Analysis Behavior 5:525–528.

Barltrop, D. 1966. The prevalence of pica. American Journal Diseases Child 112:116–123.

Bucher, B., Reykdal, B. and Albin, J. 1976. Brief restraint to control pica in retarded children. Journal Behavior Therapy Experimental Psychiatry 7:137–140.

Chatterjee, P. and Gettman, J.H. 1972. Lead poisoning: Subculture as a facilitating agent? American Journal Clinical Nutrition 25:324–330.

de la Burde, B. and Reames, B. 1973. Prevention of pica, the major cause of lead poisoning in children. American Journal Public Health 63:737–743.

Finney, J.W., Russo, D.C. and Cataldo, M.F. Reduction of pica in young children with lead poisoning. Journal Pediatric Psychology. In press.

Foxx, R.M. and Azrin, N.H. 1973. The elimination of autistic self-stimulatory behavior by overcorrection. Journal Applied Behavior Analysis 6:1–14.

Foxx, R.M. and Martin, E.D. 1975. Treatment of scavenging behavior (coprophagy and pica) by overcorrection. Behavior Research Therapy 13:153–162.

Lin Fu, J.S. 1973. Vulnerability of children to lead exposure and toxicity, New England Journal Medicine 289:1229–1233.

Lowtiz, G.H. and Suib, M.R. 1978. Generalized control of persistent thumbsucking by differential reinforcement of other behaviors. Journal Behavior Therapy Experimental Psychiatry 9:343–346.

Madden, N.A., Russo, D.C. and Cataldo, M.F. 1980a. Environmental influences on mouthing in children with lead intoxication. Journal Pediatric Psychology 5:207–216.

Madden, N.A., Russo, D.C. and Cataldo, M.F. 1980b. Behavioral treatment of pica in children with lead poisoning. Child Behavior Therapy 2:67–81.

Sachs, H., Blanksma, L.A., Murray, E. and O'Connell, M.J. 1970. Ambulatory treatment of lead poisoning: Report of 1155 cases. Pediatrics 46:389–399.

Sayre, J.W., Charney, E., Vostal, J. and Pless, I.B. 1974. House and hand dust as a potential source of childhood lead exposure. American Journal Diseases Child 127:167–170.

11. Coordination of Lead Screening, Prevention and Treatment Programs

Estelle Siker

Introduction

The lead screening, prevention and treatment programs of Connecticut reflect what can happen when there is a positive interplay between university-based research and state public health services. This paper will describe some of this research and show how it influenced the pattern of services provided by the state and local public health services.

The lead poisoning initiative in Connecticut was spearheaded by Dr. Martha Lepow and her students at the University of Connecticut Health Center. Epidemiologic studies have also been carried out at the Yale Department of Epidemiology and Public Health. Dr. Lepow's initial survey of children in the north end of Hartford, Connecticut, led to the appointment of a Governor's Task Force on Lead Poisoning. Legislation derived from the work of this Task Force now requires the reporting of lead poisoning with investigation and follow-up by local directors of health. In addition, the use and sale of lead-containing paint is now regulated, in conformance with Federal law.

Initial legislation provided funds for state laboratory personnel and supplies and a state coordinator. Dr. Lepow, working with the State Department of Health Services, the Hartford Health Department, Hartford Hospital and the Hartford Community Action Agency and some federal funds, established an ongoing lead poisoning screening program in greater Hartford. The program included public education and corrective housing action.

Among the numerous studies undertaken by Dr. Lepow and her colleagues was one assessing the role of airborne lead from auto emissions in the increased body burden of lead in an inner city area of Hartford (Lepow et al., 1974). High concentrations of lead were found in dirt and household dust. This plays a role in the increased lead burden of urban children when they mouth their dirty hands. Upon conclusion of the study, the investigators proposed elimination of lead from gasoline, a measure which has been adopted (see Chapter 8).

In another study, Cohen et al. (1973) compared the venous blood lead levels of 230 rural and 272 urban children whose mean age was 4 yr. Nine % of the rural children had laboratory evidence of undue lead absorption, as compared with 23% of the urban children. This was an important finding for it showed that even though the rural rate was lower, rural homes were also sources of indoor and outdoor leaded paint.

A more recent study was carried out through the New Haven Health Department Lead Project by Stark and Meigs from the Yale University School of Medicine, Department of Epidemiology and Public Health. (Stark, A.D. and Meigs, J.W. 1980. Personal communication). The survey was done in New Haven from 1974 to 1976 on over 8000 children drawn from all sections of the city. The children ranged in age from 1 to 6 yr and comprised 80% of this age cohort in the area. Blood leads were done and lead concentration in dwellings, soil and air were determined and classified according to socioeconomic status (SES) and census tracts. Extensive information also was collected on size and composition of families.

There was a steady increase in mean blood lead level as the SES went down; this was true of white, black and hispanic populations. The blood lead level was not related to the amount of lead available, which was essentially the same across the SES groups, but rather to family characteristics such as where and how children play and eat. White children were less likely to ingest lead than were black children, even within the same SES. The ages of 2 and 3 were found to be the most dangerous periods for lead ingestion. Study findings also confirmed the effect of season on lead ingestion, again suggesting that, if resources are limited, the summer is the best time to screen. (Diet and anemia are suspected of creating a potential for increased absorption.) The blood lead level is not just a function of the environment; there is some interaction of the child with the environment. Many parents were not aware of the implications of the behavior of the child, but once alerted, were able to control the activity. This has implications for public information and education.

Stark et al. (1978) also found a strong association between high blood lead and socioeconomic factors such as single parent and large numbers of children. Attendance in a day care program appeared to provide some protection.

Coordinated Programming

A number of disciplines are involved in lead programs at the state and local level. In Connecticut the state health services department laboratory performs a major portion of testing for lead. The remainder is done in private laboratories, clinics, hospitals and some local health departments.

In accordance with state law, lead poisoning is reported to the Preventible Disease Division, which also houses the environmental health and toxic hazards programs. The Division of Community Health Services provides personal health services such as maternal and child health and health education. After a recent reorganization aimed at improving coordination of services, all these functions are now located in the Bureau of Health Promotion and Disease Prevention.

Connecticut has 169 independent towns. At the local level, health departments work with clinics, hospitals, private physicians, public health nursing organizations and community groups. They also deal with housing administrations, since not all housing sections are under control of the local health departments. This makes coordination of health services a complex and important job.

The state employs a health educator as a state lead coordinator in the Community Health Division. This position, established in 1971 by a special appropriation from the legislature, is responsible for coordinating the various units at the state level and for promoting and assisting with education, screening and follow-up programs for 1- to 6-yr-old children throughout the state.

In the 1970's numerous mass screening programs were conducted. However, experience showed that it is difficult to maintain mass screening on an ongoing basis. It is more feasible to incorporate lead poisoning education and screening into ongoing Federally, state or locally funded programs. Outreach is used to bring the children into the health care screening and education system.

There is a variety of ongoing programs that can be used as vehicles for lead poisoning education, screening and follow-up. The March 1979 joint statement of the Bureau of Community Health Services (BCHS) and Centers for Disease Control (CDC) recommended that each of the BCHS projects and programs serving the 1- to 6-yr-old age group determine the risk in its population and, if undue absorption of lead is found, offer lead screening as part of its comprehensive services.

Title V of the Social Security Act provides formula grants to the states for Maternal and Child Health and Crippled Children's Services. In many states, state and county governments operate child health or well-baby clinics which provide primarily preventive and health supervision services to children from infancy to school entry. These clinics can also provide education and screening. For fiscal year 1979-1980, 44 (71%) of the 62 Connecticut agencies operating such clinics offered lead screening. Over 8000 lead screening tests were done, and 6.5% of those screenings revealed unacceptable body burdens of lead.

Maternity and infant care projects serve infants up to 1 yr of age, and children and youth projects provide comprehensive and continuous care for children from birth to age 21. These programs include lead screening as part of comprehensive care.

In addition to the maternal and child health programs, the Bureau of Community Health Services also funds community health centers, rural and urban health initiatives, migrant worker health programs and health maintenance organizations. Lead screening can be part of the comprehensive health services of each of these programs.

The Early and Periodic Screening, Diagnosis and Treatment Program (EPSDT) of Title XIX, is also designed to provide screening on a periodic basis and to provide follow-up, diagnosis and treatment of children from birth to age 21. Lead poisoning is one of the conditions which is reported to the federal Medicaid agency. In Connecticut, there are 154 EPSDT providers serving 3000 children monthly. Of this number, only 3.5% are tested for lead.

Child day care centers and Head Start programs can be used for educational programs for families, as sites for screening and also as resources for placement of children at risk in the home environment. In 1979 the state fielded a demonstration in which trained CETA workers went into child day care centers with a program of nutrition and dental health education for staff and parents and lead screening for the children. Of the 300 tests done, five follow-ups were required. Unfortunately, when the CETA grant ended this effort could not be continued.

The Women, Infants and Children Program (WIC) offers supplemental food for pregnant and nursing women, infants and children. It also might be a vehicle for lead screening in areas where health resources are scarce. The WIC program certifies those nutritionally at risk. It is interesting to speculate whether this program, which supplies protein, calcium, iron and vitamin C, might also offer a protection against lead absorption. (See Chapter 7.)

Finally, other health resources such as hospitals, local health departments primary care clinics and high risk clinics for children can serve as sites for lead programs.

On an annual basis, the Connecticut state laboratory reports approximately 25,000 children screened. Of this number, a consistent 10 to 15% show evidence of undue lead absorption. The majority of these children are screened through local health departments, well-child clinics and day care or Head Start programs. Additional screening is conducted as part of special events such as health fairs sponsored by civic, religious or community organizations.

The Connecticut lead program coordinator consults the state environmental health and health statistics units for information, on town housing stock and on community demographic characteristics in order to identify children presumably at risk. Laboratory reports indicate the amount of testing already done. Where indicated, the coordinator approaches the local health director, requesting the information of a local community planning group to provide continuing support for a lead poisoning program.

Once the green light is given by the planning group and the local agency, the coordinator goes directly to the resources serving children of the proper age group. The attempt is made to incorporate a lead program with existing services. Part of the coordinator's job is to provide educational programs for the staff and parents of children served by Head Start and day care. She also works with parent-teacher associations throughout the state. Personal contacts are made with child health clinics offering assistance in education, screening and follow-up according to the Federal guidelines. An education program for the staff also assists them in interpreting laboratory results.

Health fairs are another area of activity. A physician is identified to receive laboratory reports and to work with a local health director with regard to follow-up. These functions are especially helpful in identifying children not in the health system.

Several years ago Federal funds were granted to the state Department of Health Services to improve its laboratory and to five towns in Connecticut to establish programs. Two of the state's large cities still have Federal grants. Through their health departments they coordinate outreach to identify needy children and to bring them into the health care system. The communities which no longer are funded have established a system of identification of children who may have lead poisoning.

Conclusion

In Connecticut, as elsewhere, there is a lack of money and staff to do required follow-up, to collect and maintain adequate data, to provide more intensive public education and to more fully incorporate screening for lead poisoning into the health care programs that serve children at risk. This paper has shown that a network of services exists and that there is potential for coordination and funding. A key element in providing impetus for this support is the work of researchers in the academic community. More such cooperative efforts are needed.

References

Lepow, M.L., Bruckman L., Markowitz, S., Robino, R., Kapish, J. 1975. Investigations into sources of lead in the environment of urban children. Environ Res 10:415.

Lepow, M.L., Bruckman L., Rubino, R. 1974. Role of airborne lead in increased body burden of lead of Hartford children. Environ Health Persp 7:99–102.

Cohen, C.J., Bowers, G.N. and Lepow, M.L. 1973. Epidemiology of lead poisoning: A comparison between urban and rural children. JAMA 226:1430–1433.

Stark, A.D. and Meigs, J.W. 1980. Personal communication.

Stark, A.D., Meigs, J.W., Fitch, R.A. and De-Louise, E.R. 1978. Family operational co-factors in the epidemiology of childhood lead poisoning. Arch Environ Health 33:222–225.

12. Laboratory Aspects of Lead Poisoning Control

Douglas G. Mitchell

Introduction

This chapter describes some of the steps needed to ensure data quality for blood lead (PbB) and erythrocyte protoporphyrin (EP) analysis.

Historically, it has been difficult to get good PbB and EP data. Prior to 1970, PbB was the only test done, and it was carried out on a 10-ml blood sample using a dithizone extraction procedure. The sample was difficult to obtain and the analytical method required considerable skill. During 1970 to 1972 an extraction-atomic absorption procedure (Hessel, 1968) was introduced. This required 4 ml of blood and was a much easier analytical procedure. Fingerstick procedures were introduced in 1972 (Mitchell et al., 1974). These used about 60 μl of blood, which greatly facilitated sample collection. However, microprocedures demand very clean sample collection techniques and skilled analytical chemistry. About 1974, EP analysis by extraction-fluorometry (Piomelli et al., 1973) was introduced. This procedure uses only fingerstick samples and routine sample collection techniques, but it requires skilled and careful chemical analysis. In

Table 1. Selected data from the CDC PB Proficiency Testing Program, January 1979.

Method	Number of Analyses	PB Concentration in μg/dl (RSD, %)		
		High	Medium	Low
Delves cup	34	69 (9%)	41 (9%)	8 (38%)
Anodic stripping voltametry	23	70 (10%)	41 (14%)	9 (25%)

1977, the hematofluorometer was introduced. Although this instrument requires only good calibration, it is more prone to error than is extraction.

At present, PbB is most commonly determined by Delves cup atomic absorption or anodic stripping voltametry, and EP is usually determined with a hematofluorometer or by extraction.

Current Laboratory Performance

In the Center for Disease Control (CDC) PbB proficiency testing program, three samples were shipped to each participating laboratory in January, 1979. Table 1 shows the mean lead concentrations (μg/dl) and relative standard deviations (%), after rejecting extreme outliers, for laboratories using the two most popular techniques. Relative standard deviations of about 10% at the higher concentrations are excellent for an analysis of this difficulty.

Similar data for EP analyses (Table 2) also show excellent precision, although there seem to be systematic differences between the Piomelli et al. extraction procedure (1973) and the hematofluorometer.

Proficiency testing, however, evaluates laboratory performance under optimum conditions. In routine screening the data quality may be much worse.

Table 2.   Selected data from the CDC EP Proficiency Testing Program, January 1979.

Method	Number of Analyses	EP Concentration in μg/dl (RSD, %)		
		High	Medium	Low
Piomelli	33	153 (9%)	83 (11%)	26 (26%)
Hematofluorometer	86	169 (6%)	92 (6%)	20 (20%)

Procedures for Ensuring Data Quality

Sample collection is the first step in the analysis. For PbB it is probably the step most prone to error. Sweat typically contains over 100 μg Pb/dl, and dust can contain several per cent of lead. Hence, blood must be collected by a scrupulously clean technique.

Blood collectors need training and their performance must be monitored for at least the first 25 samples collected. Performance can be checked readily by

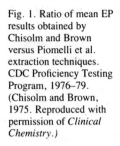

Fig. 1. Ratio of mean EP results obtained by Chisolm and Brown versus Piomelli et al. extraction techniques. CDC Proficiency Testing Program, 1976–79. (Chisolm and Brown, 1975. Reproduced with permission of *Clinical Chemistry*.)

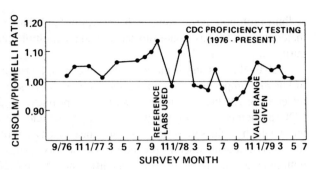

collecting two capillary tubes per patient and comparing the PbB levels. Differences of about 10 µg/dl or more between the two tubes strongly suggest a poor collection technique.

Sample storage and shipping are also important. Samples should be refrigerated until shipped and then shipped as soon as possible. Because protoporphyrin is sensitive to light, all samples for EP analysis must be stored in the dark. The extraction EP procedure and several PbB procedures are sensitive to heat and tend to give low results with old samples.

Blood Lead and Protoporphyrin Measurement Techniques

Blood lead analysis is now a mature technique. Apart from problems in handling samples noted above, the major unsolved problem with blood lead analysis is the lack of a certified standard.

With EP analysis the major problem is calibration. Figure 1 shows the results of CDC proficiency testing of two procedures from September, 1976, to May, 1979. The ratio of mean EP results by Chisolm and Brown extraction (1975) to those by Piomelli et al. extraction (1973) is plotted against time. If both procedures are either free from or subject to the same bias, the ratio will be 1.0. In fact, the two procedures have shown systematic differences of up to 15%.

This bias is due partly to a lack of pure standards. Figure 2 shows a liquid chromatogram of a widely used zinc protoporphyrin standard. The large peak is zinc protoporphyrin. The smaller peaks are porphyrin impurities, which have a fluorescence response similar but not identical to that of zinc protoporphyrin. The net result is that the concentration of the standard is not accurately known. Figure 3 (Smith et al., 1980) shows a liquid chromatogram of commercial sodium protoporphyrin using both absorption and fluorescence detectors. This material is not sold as a pure substance, and the multiple peaks confirm its lack of purity.

Analytical chemistry is based on the concept of a primary standard, a material of known composition for comparison with unknown samples. There is no such material for EP analysis. In practice, the real primary standard is performance in CDC proficiency testing programs. Laboratories choose as standard materials those which yield satisfactory performance in CDC proficiency tests. This is obviously not a satisfactory procedure. Laboratory results as a group could drift with time, as each laboratory corrects differences from CDC target values. If this occurs, it is not easily detected without a recognized primary standard. For example, an action level of 50 μg EP/dl could drift to 45 μg EP/dl with time.

The hematofluorometer is the most recent development in EP analysis. This instrument measures zinc protoporphyrin concentrations, calibrated as EP, by front-surface fluorometry on whole, untreated blood. The instrument has very obvious advantages. It does not require sample pretreatment, and allows rapid measurement to be carried out in the field. Once again, the major problem is calibration. The hematofluorometer is calibrated with a fluorescent dye slide

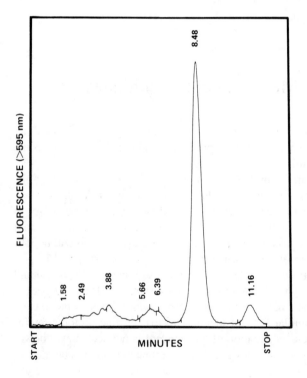

Fig. 2. Liquid chromatogram of a zinc protoporphyrin standard, using a fluorescence detector (Smith et al., 1980. Reproduced with permission of the *Journal of Chromatography*.)

which has been calibrated against human blood by the manufacturer. The instrument user cannot check the instrument directly against commercial blood standards because the instrument is less reliable with aged blood.

The only certain calibration procedure is analysis of a series of blood samples using both the hematofluorometer and an extraction technique. The hematofluorometer is used with freshly drawn blood and the extraction technique with blood

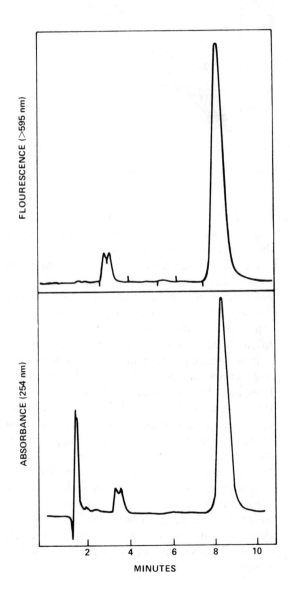

Fig. 3. Liquid chromatogram of commercial sodium protoporphyrin, using both absorption and fluorescence detectors (Smith, 1980. Reproduced with permission of the *Journal of Chromatography.*)

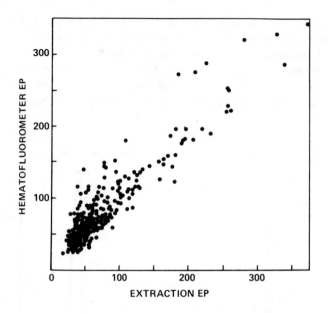

Fig. 4.
Hematofluorometer EP
levels plotted against
extraction EP levels for
fingerstick blood
samples.

up to 7 days old. Figure 4 shows a comparison of such results for a group of fingerstick samples (D.R. Doran and D.G. Mitchell, unpublished data). Ideally, the results should be on a line at 45° to the X-axis. The actual data are quite scattered, although there is less scatter with venipuncture samples, presumably because they are less sensitive to light, heat and cold. Occasional samples show gross differences between the hematofluorometer and extraction EP results. Analysis by liquid chromatography usually agrees with the extraction procedure (Smith et al., 1980). These outlying points should be rejected and a line of best fit calculated. This yields an optimum intercept of 0.0 and slope of 1.0.

In practice, the hematofluorometer may show significant bias. For example, in an experiment in the New York State Department of Health laboratory, a slope of 0.89 was obtained, indicating that the hematofluorometer read 11% too low (D.R. Doran and D.G. Mitchell, unpublished results). Hematofluorometer standards were corrected and the experiment was repeated, yielding a slope of 0.99. However, 2 mos later the slope had dropped to 0.87, indicating that the hematofluorometer was yielding results 13% too low. A less likely alternative was that the extraction procedure yielded high results.

It is strongly recommended that such calibration procedures be carried out at regular intervals, with the interval determined by the stability of the hematofluorometer. Otherwise, the instrument could yield biased data which cannot be detected easily. Satisfactory performance in proficiency testing with synthetic samples suggests, but does not guarantee, satisfactory performance with patient samples.

Conclusion

Over the past few years laboratory performance in both PbB and EP analysis has improved considerably. However, concern for data quality is essential. PbB analysis is still subject to important problems with sample collection. EP analysis by both commonly used techniques has important, although not obvious, problems with calibration. Care, vigilance and a reasonable amount of skepticism are still in order.

Acknowledgment

The author thanks Ms. D.R. Doran for assistance in preparing this manuscript and in much of the experimental work.

References

Chisolm, J.J. and Brown, D.H. 1975. Microscale photofluorometric determination of "free erythrocyte porphyrin" (Protoporphyrin IX). Clin Chem 21:1669–1681.

Hessel, D.W. 1968. A simple and rapid quantitative determination of lead in blood. Atomic Absorp Newsl 7:55.

Mitchell, D.G., Aldous, K.M. and Ryan, F.J. 1974. Mass screening for lead poisoning. New York State J Med 74:1599–1603.

Piomelli, S. Davidow, B., Guinee, V.F., Young, P. and Gay, G. 1973. The FEP (free erythrocyte porphyrins) test: A screening micromethod for lead poisoning. Pediatrics 51:254–259.

Smith, R. Doran, D., Mazur, M. and Bush, B. 1980. High-performance liquid chromatographic determination of protoporphyrin and zinc protoporphyrin in blood. J Chromatogr, 181:319–327.

13. Methods for Abating Lead Hazards in Housing

Lawrence Chadzynski

This chapter will focus on methods of abating identified lead hazards in the home environment of the child with an added body burden of lead.

Methods

Following the identification of the most probable source(s) of lead contributing to the illness of the child, an orderly but expedient process of environmental intervention should be pursued. The three major courses of action are removal of the child from the lead source, removal of the lead source and provision of a barrier between the lead source and the child. Characteristics of the specific situation will determine which strategies to employ.

Risk is important in determining the course of environmental hazard reduction. In dwellings occupied by children classified by the Center for Disease Control (CDC) as Class III or IV, especially children hospitalized or undergoing treatment, emergency repairs should be ordered immediately upon identification of the hazards. This includes instruction to the occupants and/or owners to scrape off all loose and flaking lead paint and to clean up by sweeping and wet mopping the floors and washing the walls. A simple temporary repair measure is to move a sofa to cover a small hole in the wall surface where a toddler was seen picking at and eating paint. Some inspectors carry with them a 4-in-wide roll of masking tape with which to cover immediately chipping, flaking and peeling lead-painted surfaces.

Emergency Repair Methods

Emergency repair measures are actions that will minimize exposure of the child to identified lead hazards until approved permanent repairs can be made. They include, but are not limited to, the following.

Scraping.   All peeling, chipping or flaking lead-based paint should be thoroughly scraped. All scrapings should be swept up, wrapped and sealed in some type of container and removed from the premises. For example, lead paint scrapings may be transferred to a lead smelting firm for recycling.

Sanding.   A rough grade of sandpaper should be used to sand off lead-based paint on readily accessible surfaces such as door frames, door jambs, woodwork and window sills. Safety measures for both worker and occupant are of primary importance when scraping and sanding.

Covering.   Inexpensive contact paper may be applied to all lead-based painted surfaces, especially window sills and surfaces presenting a biting edge to the child. Lead-based painted surfaces may also be covered with a material such as wallboard or plywood to prohibit easy access.

All areas on which temporary repairs have been made should be maintained daily so that they remain free of loose and flaking lead-based paint until permanent repairs are made.

Permanent Repair Methods

Permanent repairs are those of a more lasting nature, such that the lead-poisoned child, siblings or other children are no longer exposed to the lead hazard. All lead-based painted surfaces that are in a cracking, peeling, chipping, or flaking condition must be removed or covered. This also is true of lead-based painted surfaces accessible to children.

The method or process used for the removal of lead-based paint should not present a hazard to the health of the workers or occupants from fumes, dust, vapors or liquids by inhalation or absorption through the skin and mucous membranes. When lead paint is removed from surfaces, hazards may arise from the lead paint which is being removed or from toxic materials used in the removal, especially in inadequately ventilated areas.

Simply painting over lead-based painted surfaces is an unacceptable abatement method. The most common acceptable methods of removing lead paint from surfaces are scraping and sanding, removing paint with solvents, heating and covering.

Scraping and Sanding.   Scraping or sanding requires the most labor. The process results in large amounts of lead dust and particles being placed in the air which may, in the process, result in a lead hazard to the worker or occupants. Workmen should wear respirators approved by the U.S. Bureau of Mines. Safety goggles and protective clothing are recommended also. All loose, peeling or flaking paint should be scraped off and the remainder sanded or scraped down to the base material. The surface should then be patched, sealed and repainted with non-lead coatings. Tarps or plastic floor coverings should be used to collect the waste and residue caused by the operation. These should then be removed from the premises and disposed of in a safe manner. The inhalation of low concentrations of lead particles over a long period of time can result in lead poisoning.

Removing Paint with Solvent.   Solvents evaporate readily and can be inhaled. Solvents and paint removers can also be absorbed through the skin.

Liquid paint removers are usually used on small areas such as windowsills, doors and woodwork. The solvent softens the paint which may then be removed by scraping. Some skill is required in using solvents and there is considerable danger if they are not used in the manner prescribed on the label instructions. Solvents are extremely flammable, can burn the skin and should be used with the utmost caution in a well ventilated area. Impervious gloves should also be worn. A respirator designed for protection against organic vapors is recommended when liquid paint removers are used. Floor surfaces should be protected from spillage of residue-containing solvents.

Heating.   The removal of leaded paint by heating will produce lead fumes which are toxic if inhaled in small concentrations. This danger can be minimized if the heating device is used only to soften the paint so that it can be scraped off, thereby preventing the paint from igniting. Heating is accomplished by use of a gas-fired torch, infrared lamp or electric heat gun. A heating device should be used only by a person experienced in its use. He should be aware of the potential danger of fire by igniting the painted surface and adjacent wall areas. A respirator approved by the U.S. Bureau of Mines for fumes should be used to prevent the inhalation of lead fumes. In addition, protective eye glasses and clothing should be worn when infra-red units are used. Although heating is frequently used for removal of lead paint, it is recognized as the most hazardous method from the standpoint of the dangers of igniting the building and poisoning the workers and occupants from lead fumes. This method of removal should be used only with strict adherence to safety precautions. As an added precaution a workable fire extinguisher should be handy.

Covering.   This relatively inexpensive method is the safest and most acceptable of environmental lead hazard reduction techniques. Wallboard, hardboard, plywood paneling, vinyl wall covering, jute fabrics, fiberglass or a similar durable material is applied to cover the walls. The material is affixed by nailing, cementing or gluing so that it cannot be removed or damaged by a small child or by continued normal wear and use. The application must be vermin-proof. If it is used in common areas of multiple dwelling units it must be fire resistant or retardant. Moldings should be installed at junctions of walls and ceiling and walls and floor to prevent loosening of materials. Local fire laws should be reviewed for restrictions in the use of wall covering materials.

All lead-based painted woodwork that is readily accessible to the child should be stripped or scraped down to bare wood or other base material. Woodwork should be primed and painted with non-leaded paint only after the removal of old paint has been verified by the investigator. Consideration may be given to the replacement of lead-painted woodwork such as windowsills, moldings, baseboards, doors and door jambs as an alternative abatement method.

Loose, leaded putty must be removed and replaced with non-leaded putty.

The ingestion of lead-enriched soil found around the housing structure and its outbuildings can contribute significant amounts of lead to the intake of the child. This is especially true in summer months and in areas with more temperate climates. Abatement is achieved by turning the soil over, sodding with grass, removing heavily contaminated soil or paving with concrete.

Lead-based painted walls and ceiling surfaces that are tight or intact, regardless of their lead content, are not required to be deleaded. The owner or landlord should, however, be notified that the painted surfaces contain lead and that as long as they are maintained in a tight or intact condition they do not present a hazard. However, all readily accessible surfaces must be abated whether the lead-based paint is intact or not (Chadzynski and Benvenuti, 1978).

The foregoing lead hazard abatement methodology represents the current state of the art. It is hoped a more effective and efficient lead paint hazard removal method will be developed. Until then, lead hazard reduction activities should focus on a site-specific approach to their abatement.

Safety of Workers and Occupants during the Abatement Process

It is important to note that whatever method is used for the removal of leaded paint, both the occupants and the workers should be protected from exposure to lead stemming from the abatement process itself.

The abatement method used should not present a hazard to the health of the workers or occupants from fumes, dust, vapors or liquids by ingestion, inhalation or absorption through the skin, mucous membranes and alimentary and respiratory tracts. During the deleading process, hazards may arise either from the lead which is being removed or from toxic materials used in the removal process especially if the work is done in inadequately ventilated areas.

Debris Containment

Paint removal workers and contractors should demonstrate concern for lead debris containment. Debris containment implies that preventive measures be taken to minimize the dispersion of leaded-paint flakes and dust generated during the deleading procedure. For example, a relatively new device on the market, called a Beadpack Paint and Rust Removal Machine, controls the spent beads and removed paint debris, thereby precluding any cleanup or contamination of the working environment. Also on the market are commercial vacuum cleaners with attached filters that prevent lead debris from becoming airborne.

Newspapers or plastic or canvas tarps should be used to cover the floors just as one would do prior to painting to avoid soiling the floors and furniture. Upon completion of the work, all floors and walls should be vacuumed and wet washed to remove any residual lead.

Whenever possible, the occupants should seek temporary shelter during the deleading process. At a minimum, interior work should be planned so as to delead one room at a time. By confining the work area to one part of the house or apartment, dispersion of an exposure to lead can be minimized.

Safety Devices

In the discussion of abatement methods safety devices and precautions were stressed in relation to each specific abatement method. This section presents a more detailed description of safety factors.

In addition to the concern that the work area be well ventilated, there are other precautions and safety devices that should be employed by the workers to minimize their exposure to lead hazards. The safety devices vary by the deleading method selected. Workers and occupants must be protected from dust, fumes, vapors and liquids.

Scraping and Sanding.   This method of leaded paint removal creates large amounts of dust which becomes airborne and can settle throughout the premises if not contained. It is important that dust collectors be used along with this process and that the work area be well ventilated. Respirators should be worn by the workers in addition to protective clothing and goggles.

Removing Paint with Solvents.   The concern here is for toxic vapors, burns, fire and explosion from the paint remover formulation. Many paint removers contain methylene chloride, which is highly volatile. Its vapors, if inhaled, can cause illness and death. In using this method, it is again important to stress that the work area should be well ventilated. Protective clothing, gloves and goggles should be worn.

Heating.   Concern here is with fire and fumes. It is important that the workmen wear respirators and protective clothing, goggles and gloves. The surface should be heated to the point that the paint is softened just enough to remove it with a scraper.

The Childhood Lead-Based Paint Poisoning Prevention Act of 1973 requires removal of existing lead-based paint in dwellings where children under 6 yrs of age reside. This regulation has increased the number of workers employed in the deleading of homes. Many of the firms engaged in this type of work are small, independent enterprises and may not be sophisticated enough to monitor employee lead levels or to require that their employees wear protective equipment. Moreover, they may not recognize the need for the containment of lead residue. Consequently, paint removal employees are at risk of becoming lead poisoned. In this regard, it is important that investigators generate a concern for protection of lead workers and for the containment of lead debris produced through the abatement process.

Disposal of Lead

The Environmental Protection Agency (EPA) is concerned with the safe and proper disposal of lead residue. However, until the EPA issues regulations, the following approaches are used in disposing of lead debris.

Following the deleading process, all lead debris should be put in plastic bags, sealed and taken to a sanitary land fill or to a lead smelter. One western city has made arrangements with a local lead smelter to accept lead debris from its lead hazard abatement program for safe disposal.

Lead debris should not be disposed of in any manner whereby lead can be reintroduced into public or private waterways or water supplies. Lead debris should not be incinerated in open fires or dumps.

Summary

In summary, this chapter has evolved from program experience. The lead hazard abatement methods presented here represent current efforts to delead the environment of children who have an added body burden of lead.

One of the fundamental environmental objectives of the Detroit, Michigan, program is to not close a case of lead poisoning until the lead level of the affected child has returned to normal. This is accomplished when the sources of lead causing the problem are identified and abated. Therefore, it is of primary concern that lead investigators have a working knowledge of the methods of lead hazard abatement and their implicit problems and a commitment to remove lead hazards expeditiously. Under no circumstances should a child with an identified source of lead poisoning continue to be exposed to the lead hazard causing the condition.

References

Chadzynski, L. 1980. Finding the Source of Lead. In Low Level Lead Exposure: The Clinical Implications of Current Research. H.L. Needleman Ed. New York: Raven Press. 239–251.

Chadzynski, L. and Benvenuti, A. 1978. Investigator's Manual for Environmental Lead Hazard Identification and Abatement. Detroit Health Department.

U.S. Department of Health, Education and Welfare 1978. Preventing Lead Poisoning in Young Children. A Statement by the Center for Disease Control. Public Health Service, Bureau of State Services, Environmental Health Services Division, Atlanta.

14. Some Problems Associated with the Environmental Phases of a Childhood Lead Poisoning Prevention Program

Walter J. Sobolesky

Introduction

The city of Philadelphia has been directly involved in the control of childhood lead poisoning since 1950. Until 1970, the program was directed primarily at identifying the lead source only in symptomatic cases of childhood lead poisoning and in cases reported to the Philadelphia Department of Public Health by private physicians who were concerned about the continued exposure of the child to lead. From 1950 to 1966, investigations were made of the environment of the child and, eventually, orders were issued to the property owner to remove the lead source, primarily lead-based paint. Enforcement of orders was extremely difficult and resulted in long delays because the department had no specific regulations on removal of lead hazards.

In 1966, regulations were passed and the City Code was amended, permitting the department to issue orders for removal of lead sources from a child reported to have lead poisoning. Until 1970, the department continued to investigate only reported cases of lead poisoning and enforced the ordinance, if needed, through orders of a Court of Equity. These procedures, while effective, resulted in extremely long delays since the courts did not consider lead poisoning cases a priority over criminal cases.

During these years, removal of the lead hazard was done by the property owner or a private contractor and there was no attempt by the department to determine the method used or the degree of exposure to workers and members of the household during the abatement.

In 1970, the Department received a large grant from the Model Cities Program to implement a comprehensive program to control childhood lead poisoning. The grant allowed the department to hire personnel to remove lead-based paint from dwelling units occupied by children under 6 yr of age, providing the department indicated the lead-based paint was a health hazard.

Implementation of Abatement Techniques

While the comprehensive program included screening, medical management of children, environmental investigations and reduction of lead hazards at no cost to residents of the Model Cities area, the safety and health of abatement employees and occupants of the dwelling units was a major concern of the Department.

Various methods for removing lead based paint from woodwork were investigated and tested during the early stages of the program. Within the city, lead-based paint was only found in woodwork, while walls and ceilings were generally not painted. The latter surfaces were usually covered with wallpaper and, therefore, did not require abatement. This was an extremely beneficial circumstance since abatement costs to the program would have been increased greatly if walls and ceilings required abatement.

First attempts to utilize electric heating units (an electric coil within a metal box frame) to remove the hazard proved to be very inefficient and very costly because these units were cumbersome and time-consuming. In addition, they required electricity which, while available in the homes being abated, was usually from a fuse box system with approximately 15 amps available on the line. The electric units, therefore, would cause blowing of fuses, resulting in considerable downtime in worker productivity. The electric units also resulted in numerous cracked window panes, especially in cold weather, because the heat could not be regulated either by temperature or area of distribution, i.e., heat could not be pin-pointed.

Other methods to remove lead-based paint included torch lamps, infrared lamps and the acetylene torch. The first two also proved to be inefficient and had several disadvantages with no apparent advantages to safeguard the health of our employees and to provide a measure of safety to the occupants or the property itself. Some of the disadvantages included excessive heat, danger of eye damage and burning of paint particles. In addition, the cumbersome apparatus caused operational fatigue and increased operational costs because productivity was lessened and equipment breakdowns were common.

Based on overall performance of the abatement crews using these three, the acetylene torch was the method of choice, in spite of its potential as a fire hazard and the generation of lead fumes while burning off the lead-based paint. From 1971 to 1975, abatements performed by project personnel utilized the acetylene torch method. Arrangements were made with a local smelting firm to have all lead paint residue resulting from abatements delivered to the smelter and recycled, allowing the firm to reclaim the small amount of lead present.

In 1973, the project director reviewed literature on the use of "heat guns" for drying glassware and utensils and for softening glass tubing and plastic piping. The thought occurred that this equipment might be used for softening paint (rather than burning it), thereby greatly reducing the fire hazard and, possibly, the exposure to lead fumes of abatement personnel.

Better abatement methods were needed since claims against the city for property damage due to fire were not uncommon. In addition, blood lead levels of abatement personnel were rising even though employees were required to wear canister-type respirators approved for lead fumes and mists while burning off lead-based paint. Early studies on lead levels of abatement personnel indicated high lead levels resulting from abatement by acetylene torch. Table 1 shows the abnormal air lead levels found with this method.

Trial studies of the flameless electric heat guns quickly indicated that this equipment had many advantages over the other methods. It produced cleaner abated surfaces with little or no charring of woodwork and adjacent surfaces, eliminated window pane breakage, generated no discomforting heat, virtually eliminated fire hazards and decreased the likelihood of generating lead fumes. In addition, the operator could wear more comfortable respirators, the equipment was easy to use and the overall fatigue problem of the employees was lessened. Disadvantages in the use of the heat guns were the longer time needed to remove the lead-based paint, the need for an electrical source other than regular house current (which was unsuitable) and a slight increase in abatement costs. How-

Table 1.   Lead levels present in air in work areas while burning off lead-based paint by acetylene torch.

| | | Personnel | |
	Adjacent to Work Area	Burning Off	Sanding and Cleaning
Filters exposed (N)	69	75	49
Mean lead level ($\mu g/m^3$)	138	115	580
Range ($\mu g/m^3$)	0–1283	0–1040	0–6400
Over TLV of 200 $\mu g/m^3$ (%)*	22	19	45

*Exposure standard at time of study; TLV, threshold limit value.

Table 2.   Lead levels present in air in work areas while removing lead-based paint by heat gun.

	Adjacent to Work Areas	Personnel	
		Stripping	Sanding and Clean Up
Filters exposed (N)	30	13	4
Mean lead level (μg/m^3)	9	8	0.0
Range (μg/m^3)	0–76	0–30	0.0
Over TLV of 200 μg/m^3 (%)	0.0	0.0	0.0

ever, when these were measured against the advantages, it was decided that this method would be the one of choice.

Studies on air lead levels were conducted during abatement procedures when the heat guns were in use. The results of these early studies are shown in Table 2. Comparing these results with those in Table 1, it is obvious that the lead in the air in working areas where the heat guns were used was significantly less than when acetylene torches were used.

In compliance with OSHA requirements for occupational exposure to lead, employees are regularly monitored while abating lead-based paint hazards. This includes air monitoring (ambient samples, breathing zone samples, air samples adjacent to the employee and air samples in an adjacent room where no deleading is occurring) and a medical surveillance program which includes blood lead levels of all abatement workers at least every 3 mos and more frequently on any employee whose blood lead level reaces 40 μg/dl. Any worker whose blood lead level is 50 μg/dl or greater must be removed until his blood lead level recedes below 30 μg/dl.

It is important to stress the need for a strong local ordinance to support an environmental control program related to lead exposure. As indicated previously, initial regulations by the city were passed in 1966. These regulations required amending, however, since federal standards were reduced twice during the years when the Philadelphia project received its first lead grant in 1972. In 1978, the amended city code established the allowable content of lead in dried paint as 0.06% by weight and also established that lead content of 0.7 mg/cm^2 or greater on dried film could be a health hazard to any child under 6 yr of age. Both standards were consistent with the Federal act and the project began using these standards in April, 1978.

In addition, the amended Code allowed the City to abate a lead hazard if the property owner did not comply with orders issued by the Department of Public Health. The property owner was then billed for the costs involved. If these were not paid within 30 days, a lien in the amount of the bill was placed against the property. This was an extremely important part of the new code since it virtually eliminated long delays in court proceedings and allowed the removal of lead hazards in urgent risk cases within 48 hr.

The authority and capability of the Philadelphia project to abate lead hazards quickly is not found in other childhood lead poisoning prevention projects. Furthermore, federal standards have not been adopted by many projects. Different communities have different standards. As a result, what constitutes a lead hazard in Philadelphia may not be a hazard in New York or Chicago.

Funding sources for environmental control, especially hazard reduction, are almost non-existent in most projects. Federal funding continues to decrease while operational costs increase. In addition, there are strict limitations on the use of funds for hazard reduction unless there is a well defined emergency with a confirmed case of lead poisoning. The limitations exclude the abatement of almost all high and moderate risk children with lead toxicity so that most programs experience long delays in lead hazards reduction. Community Development funds have been granted to the Philadelphia project for the environmental aspects of the project, both inspection and abatement. The abatement phase is restricted, however, to dwelling units where the income of the property owner is within the guidelines established by the U.S. Department of Housing and Urban Development. The current income levels accepted by HUD are shown in Table 3.

Funds received from the Department of Housing and Urban Development (HUD) can be used to abate lead hazards defined by local ordinance and need not be restricted to conditions defined in HUD regulations. Tight surfaces, e.g., those that are not cracked, peeling or chipping, regardless of the lead content, are not considered a violation of HUD regulations but can be abated if the local ordinance requires their removal.

Another area of concern is the inspection of the home environment for lead hazards. In the Philadelphia project, environmental investigations are not initiated solely on the results of a screening capillary blood test but after the screening tests have been confirmed by a venous blood sample or by a repeat capillary blood test in children initially designated as Class II (moderate risk). These procedures do result in slight delays in making inspections of dwelling units, but our experience indicates that the delays are of less concern than is the issuing of orders to property owners based on false positive screening tests.

Table 3.   HUD guidelines for income levels.

Family Size	Gross Income Level
1	$11,800
2	13,500
3	15,200
4	16,900
5	17,950
6	19,000
7	20,050
8	21,100

All dwelling units occupied by children with confirmed lead toxicity are inspected using the portable x-ray analyzer. Although the instrument is fairly accurate when in good working condition, it needs daily evaluation and frequently breaks down. Because of the low standard of 0.7 mg/cm^2, this instrument must be calibrated at least daily and sometimes after every inspection, due to its sensitivity to factors such as temperature and shock. The use of this instrument by the project is acceptable to the Philadelphia Courts, making further sampling of painted surfaces for wet chemistry analysis unnecessary. However, projects using a portable x-ray analyzer should have a backup instrument because of the downtime resulting from instrument malfunction and repair. In addition, projects should have at their disposal an XL-1 unit to measure lead content in one layer of paint on a given surface. The XL-1 can be used to verify the claim of a property owner that he has removed the lead hazard down to the bare wood and has repainted with lead-free paint. Without this instrument, a subsequent inspection with the XL-3 analyzer could result in another order being issued for removal of the newly applied lead-free paint because this analyzer would record lead-based paint residue remaining in the porous surfaces after removal.

Another area of concern is the availability of lead-based paint in retail hardware or paint stores. It should not be assumed that because Federal law prohibits the manufacturing of lead-based paint that there is none for sale. Routine inspection of retail outlets in Philadelphia continues to find lead-based paint, especially in stores which advertise special paint sales. These stores often purchase huge lots of old paint at very low prices from outlets that are going out of business. They then offer this paint at extremely low cost to the consumer. The Philadelphia ordinance allows the department to condemn such paint on the spot and to order its removal to approved land fills or other approved methods of disposal. Excellent cooperation has been received from manufacturers in getting this type of paint off the market.

Other Possible Sources of Lead

While most projects concerned with the control of childhood lead poisoning are familiar with air, dust, dirt and food as contributory sources of lead to children at risk, attention must also be given to the occupation of the parents or other members of the family. Individuals employed in industries that utilize lead can bring home significant amounts of lead on their clothing, adding to the total exposure of the child to lead. For example, policemen who spend time in indoor pistol ranges expose their clothing and themselves to lead fumes.

Another source of exposure may be a result of the energy problem. In many homes, increasing fuel costs have resulted in the use of wood stoves or coal burning stoves for heat. Old wood containing paint may be used as the heat source in many homes, especially in those where a coal stove is the only source of heat.

Conclusion

The environmental phases of any childhood lead poisoning control program are by far the most complex and most difficult to control. However, funding for a comprehensive program is a continued source of frustration to project managers. The need for instrumentation, abatement personnel, supplies and expensive equipment cannot be met if the Federal funds for environmental control are severely restricted. Projects must continue to request funding for these program needs both from existing funding sources and from other areas such as Community Development Funds, General Revenue Sharing Funds, CETA-funded programs and state or local sources.

All programs must have a strong legal basis to implement an enforcement policy and thereby eliminate delays in lead hazard reduction.

The Philadelphia project has implemented the use of heat guns as a safe and effective method of removing lead-based paint from interior and exterior surfaces. While the cost of abatement using the new method is somewhat greater than that of other methods, it is cheaper by far than jeopardizing employees and exposing inhabitants of homes to excessive lead concentrations produced by other methods of abatement. If the costs for institutionalizing a child while the lead hazard is being reduced are considered, then the utilization of the heat gun is acceptable.

15. Lead Contaminated Housedust: Hazard, Measurement and Decontamination

Christopher R. Milar and Paul Mushak

Introduction

Traditional clinical thinking has been that pediatric plumbism results from the ingestion of lead-based paint, usually as chips from peeling or chalking surfaces in older, deteriorating housing. The extensive efforts of clinicians such as Chisolm have led to a sizeable body of data characterizing the exposure environment and the constellation of adverse clinical effects produced.

More recently, however, lead in housedust has also been recognized as a potentially significant lead exposure source for children (Sayre et al., 1974; Environmental Protection Agency (EPA), 1977). Three sources of lead in housedust are sedimentation from peeling or chalking paint and from certain types of leaded paint removal procedures, fallout from automotive emissions and industrial sources in the proximity of the housing. Contributions of lead to housedust from industrial activities can be of two types, direct or primary, as in the case of emission fallout, and indirect or secondary, as in the case of a lead worker transporting the element in some fashion to the residential setting.

There have been five reports of secondary exposure of children to lead from industrial sources (Baker et al., 1977; Center for Disease Control (CDC), 1977; Dolcourt et al., 1978; Rice et al., 1978; Watson et al., 1978) where lead appeared in the home from work clothing worn by employees who handled lead.

The normal hand-to-mouth activity of young children permitted the ingestion of sufficient quantities of lead to result in elevated body burdens.

Over the past several years, a prospective study of the pediatric population first described by Dolcourt et al. (1978) has been carried out. This chapter describes one segment of this study, i.e., techniques for assessing the exposure of and behavioral effects on children exposed to housedust lead as well as the evolution and validation of dust lead decontamination methods. While the primary concern was children secondarily exposed to workplace lead, the study approaches and results are applicable to other sources of lead in housedust. The objectives of the study were to develop a methodology to assess accurately the lead content in housedust, to identify the relationship between dust lead level and an index of human exposure or biological effect and to develop and verify methods for decontamination of living areas with unacceptable levels of lead in housedust.

Obviously, any assessment of the hazard to young children of lead in housedust has to embrace the total activity environment of that child. Sayre et al. (1974) and Lepow et al. (1975) used paper towels and self-adhesive labels to sample window sills and bare floor areas. These techniques measure only a segment of the total contact environment. Few studies have attempted to assess carpeting as an exposure medium for the young child. Because many homes have carpeting and because it is usual to confine the activity area of a child to the carpeted central area of a floor, levels of dust lead in carpeting must be obtained for a meaningful exposure profile. Dolcourt et al. (1978) noted collection of dust samples from carpeting with an eye to detecting "hot spots," while the CDC study (1977) employed wet vacuuming to remove dust lead. To our knowledge, no one has attacked systematically the problem of carpeting contamination by dust lead in terms of the most reliable removal method(s), the best method of expressing content and correlation of regional analysis of carpet areas with measures such as elevated blood lead and erythrocyte protoporphyrin (EP).

Materials and Methods

Dust Sampling

The dust collection apparatus used in the study involves vacuum-assisted dry sampling. This consists of a lead-free plastic funnel connected via plastic tubing to a Gelman filter holder containing a pre-weighed 25 mm Gelman glass fiber filter for sample collection. A vacuum line from a Pro-Vac commercial vacuum cleaner is attached to the other port of the filter holder to assist in dust collection. At the end of a sampling period, the holder is disconnected and wrapped with parafilm known to have no surface lead contamination. The holders are carefully opened in the laboratory and the sample and filter weighed to give a net sample weight.

Regional sampling was carried out within a grid defined by the use of 1 m by 0.5 m wooden frame divided into equal 10-cm segments by wires. Two adjacent grids, covering an aggregate area of 1 m sq were sampled with one pass of 10 sec per grid frame. This controlled sample yielded two measures of lead, concentration as parts per million and concentration of lead expressed as micrograms per square meter ($\mu g/m^2$).

Lead Determinations

The lead content of the weighed dust samples was determined by flameless atomic absorption spectrometry using an acid-leaching technique which is a variation of the method recommended by the EPA for lead in air sampler filters (EPA, 1977). Thus, filters were heated to near boiling in dilute nitric acid, the leachate was transferred to a volumetric flask and the glass fiber filter and remaining residue were reheated with low-lead deionized water and transferred. After dilution to mark, the analytes could be diluted further if necessary with 1 N acid. (In cases of high lead contamination, extensive dilution may be necessary.) Quantitation was by the method of additions, which minimizes matrix effects.

Blood lead determinations in the children were carried out using low lead B-D Vacutainer tubes and lead measurement by atomic absorption spectrometry using the flame Delves Cup microanalysis with the variation of Ediger and Coleman (1972), i.e., the samples were preignited to destroy organic matter at a position accurately determined to avoid lead loss. The proficiency testing program of the CDC for blood lead uses the same technique.

Table 1.   Blood lead levels of children and concentration of lead in housedust, April, 1978.

Child	Age (mos)	PbB	EP	Housedust (ppm)
NL*	24	58	103	
ML*	50	55	36	1701
JL	34	49	30	
LC*	23	40	45	970
CC	59	20	55	
TW	45	40	42	7171
BL	28	49	149	
SL	28	54	130	2462
CL	45	40	20	

*Previously hospitalized for chelation.

Other Measurements

Erythrocyte protoporphyrin levels were determined using a Buchler hematofluo-rometer with correction for codetermined hematocrit.

Results and Discussion

Decontamination Procedures

Table 1 shows that dust samples for the homes of the initial sample of children averaged between 970 and 7171 ppm of lead in the housedust. In all but one instance, the children evidenced increased blood lead levels. The blood lead levels presented in the table are not the highest previous level, but represent determinations made about the time of the dust sampling. Three of the children had previously been hospitalized for chelation. At the time the samples were taken the mother of only one child (TW) was still employed in a lead-related industry. Examination of the homes of these families revealed no pre-existing lead source from the water supply, house paint or airborne sources.

The initial effort to decontaminate the homes was to use commercial carpet cleaning equipment. All rugs were vacuumed using a power carpet beater. They were then steam cleaned using a commercial Steamex® cleaner with the recommended water-detergent mixture. All uncarpeted floors were swept. They were then mopped twice, first with a Calgon® mixture of 1 lb/5 gal H_2O and then with a clear water rinse. The results of this procedure were less than satisfactory and indicated little change in the concentration of lead in the housedust of these homes. Two explanations for this are possible. The first explanation is that the level of lead in the housedust was reduced, but that the sampling procedure was inadequate to reveal the reduction. The second explanation is that the decontamination procedure was ineffective in removing lead from the homes of these children. In an attempt to improve the effectiveness of the decontamination procedure, both the sampling procedure and the decontamination procedure were changed.

The sampling procedure employed initially reports lead in housedust in terms of parts per million. Such a measure reflects concentration, but in a way that is also determined by the total collectible dust content. Thus, even though the decontamination procedure might have reduced the overall quantity of lead in the environment of the child, the extent of reduction was confounded by variation in total dust content. Put a simpler way, the concentration of lead in the housedust expressed as parts per million (ppm) reflects the amount of nonlead dust and dirt, i.e., the cleanliness of the site, as much as it does the lead content. For example, if two fixed reference areas of a carpet had the same total collectible lead content, but one area had twice the total collectible dust, a marked difference of two in lead concentrations would be determined, all other factors being equal. Thus, the concentration reading would vary with both removable lead content and the relative cleanliness of the carpet. Measuring lead content per unit area, however, is independent of the amount of nonlead dust and is a clearer measure of decontamination efforts. Furthermore, comparison of lead content in both ways also provides a relative measure of within home and between home cleanliness. This rationale prompted the change to a regional sample collected under controlled conditions that would reflect both parts per million and lead content per unit area ($\mu g/m^2$). The grid procedure of measuring a standard floor area for a precise period of time produces such a sample.

To improve the decontamination procedure, a Calgon® solution (1 lb/5 gal H_2O) was used in the Steamex® carpet cleaner. This solution was applied to both carpeted and uncarpeted surfaces. Twenty-four hours later these surfaces were then cleaned using commercial cleaning solvents in the recommended concentration. Calgon® was chosen because it is a readily available product of low toxicity that would mobilize the lead. Calgon® can be purchased from any grocery store and has a toxicity rating of 2 (Gleason et al., 1969), making it mildly toxic to non-toxic.

In order to evaluate the effectiveness of this sampling and decontamination procedure, a 12 by 15 ft carpeted room was divided into quadrants. Two of the quadrants were steam cleaned using Calgon® followed by detergent cleaning 24 hr later. The other two quadrants were cleaned using commercial detergent followed by another detergent cleaning 24 hr later. Figure 1 shows that the latter cleaning procedure was relatively ineffective, resulting in only a 12% reduction. The Calgon®-detergent cleaning, however, resulted in a 61% decrease in the concentration of lead in the housedust. The overall quantity of lead ($\mu g/m^2$) was similarly affected. In Figure 2 it can be seen that the detergent-detergent cleaning procedure resulted in a 38% reduction of lead, while the Calgon®-detergent reduced the lead by 91%. In other homes we have decontaminated, the reduction

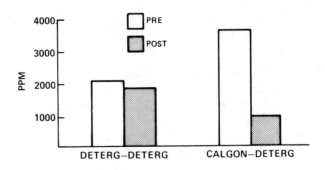

Fig. 1. Relative effectiveness of two decontamination procedures in reducing lead content of house dust measured in parts per million.

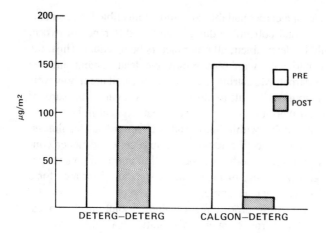

Fig. 2. Relative effectiveness of two decontamination procedures in reducing lead content of housedust measured in $\mu g/m^2$.

in concentration ranges from 30 to 50%, while the decrease in quantity of lead averages 60%. Our explanation is that Calgon® does not actually dissolve the lead but coats the particulate surface with phosphate or polyphosphate groups, reducing electrostatic interactions with carpeted surfaces and permitting easier subsequent removal by detergent. Calgon® is sodium hexa metaphosphate.

While we have been decontaminating homes of lead dust, it was possible to observe the effects of decontamination on the blood lead levels of the children. In all cases, reduction of the lead content of housedust resulted in an almost immediate decline in the lead burden of the children. An example of this is Brian, a 22-mo-old child with a blood lead (PbB) of 52 and an EP of 77 on initial screening. The initial dust sampling found his home grossly contaminated with lead. Figure 3 shows the concentration of lead in the housedust over a 10-mo period. The decontamination procedures were carried out in May, July and December, substantially reducing the concentration of lead. The middle portion of Figure 3 shows the change in the overall quantity of lead in the housedust for the same period. The change in the blood lead level of the child over the same period is presented in the bottom portion of Figure 3. Significant declines in the lead level of the child occurred between May and July and between November and January following the decontamination procedures.

The actual decontamination procedure used is as follows.

1. Sweep all uncarpeted areas. Where leaded paint is the source, it is advisable to vacuum these sites rather than re-entrain the dust into the air by sweeping.
2. If the carpet is not wall to wall, move it and vacuum underneath. Vacuuming is preferable to sweeping.
3. Replace all air conditioning and furnace filters.
4. Dissolve 1 lb of Calgon® in 5 gal of hot water.

5. Using the steam cleaner, clean all carpet and uncarpeted areas with the Calgon® solution. If the carpet is not wall to wall, the area beneath the carpet must also be cleaned. If the carpet is reversible both sides should be cleaned.
6. Twenty-four hours later, repeat the cleaning using the recommended detergent mixed in hot water in the proportions recommended by the cleaning unit manufacturers.

The study data demonstrate that this procedure is effective in reducing both the concentration and overall quantity of lead in the home environments of children.

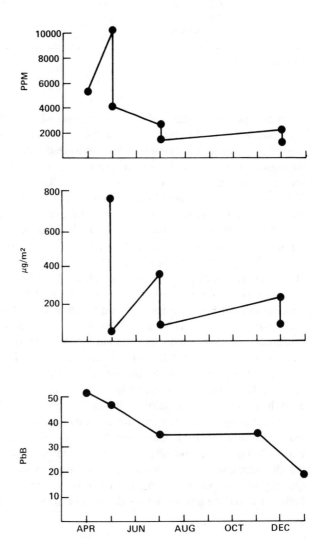

Fig. 3. Lead content of housedust measured in both parts per million and $\mu g/m^2$ over a 10-mos period. Decontamination procedures were carried out in May, July and December. The bottom portion shows the decline in the blood lead level (PbB) of the child over the same period.

Table 2.   Housedust lead levels (PPM) before and after cleaning of contaminated homes, April, 1978.

Family	Type of Surface	Before Cleanup	After Dry Vacuuming	After Cleanup
HL	Carpet-braided	1780	830	1135
	Tile	1152	—	1096
	Tile	882	—	378
	Tile	2991	—	28
MC	Carpet-loose	1205	1296	1629
	Carpet-loose	1544	2637	2254
	Carpet-tight	162	—	476
VW	Carpet-short shag	11,148	10,303	6565
	Carpet-short shag	4393	4780	4105
	Carpet-short shag	5971	*	4001
SL	Tile	1693	—	957
	Carpet-tight	*	—	2748
	Carpet-rag	3231	—	2166

*Sampling problem.

Another purpose of the study was to establish what levels of lead in housedust constitute a hazard to children. Figure 4 shows the relationship between the concentration of lead in housedust and blood lead levels of 17 children between the ages of 1.5 and 4 yr who were exposed secondarily to lead from industrial sources. The average concentration of lead in the housedust was slightly over 3000 ppm and the average blood lead level for these children was 44 μg/dl. The control children were same-aged children not exposed to lead from either industrial sources or lead-based paint. These children had an average blood lead of 18 μg/dl and the concentration of lead in the housedust of their homes was approximately 250 ppm. From these data and those of Baker et al. (1977), it seems that 1000 ppm represents the level at which children evidence increased lead absorption. In this sample of secondarily exposed children, the correlation between concentration of lead in housedust and blood lead level approached but did not reach significance. This seems to be because the concentrations of lead in housedust were lower than those found by Baker et al. (1977). However, this study sample does compare to the lower end of the Baker et al. sample and represents the point at which children begin to evidence increased lead burden resulting from lead-contaminated housedust. At the present time there are not enough samples from a sufficiently wide range of children to determine the overall quantity of lead per unit surface area ($\mu g/m^2$) in the home environment that constitutes a hazard. Clinically, however, when the concentration exceeds either 1000 ppm or 50 $\mu g/m^2$, we feel that a definite hazard exists to children and that decontamination of the home environment is indicated. We also feel that the quantity of lead per unit area ($\mu g/m^2$) in the home environment is a sensitive indicator of hazard and we are continuing our efforts to refine this measure.

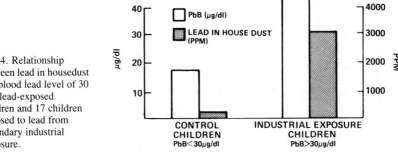

Fig. 4. Relationship between lead in housedust and blood lead level of 30 non-lead-exposed children and 17 children exposed to lead from secondary industrial exposure.

Summary

Lead in housedust can be a serious hazard to young children. Historically, it has been neglected in abatement attempts. To provide safe environments for children, it is necessary to eliminate lead contaminated housedust as well as lead-based paints in controlling lead exposure.

If in our zeal to remove lead-based paints we fail to clean up after ourselves, we could be increasing the quantity of bioavailable lead in the child's environment. Through normal hand-to-mouth activity young children can ingest sufficient amounts of leaded housedust to result in increased lead burden. The present research has presented a method of sampling to evaluate possible hazards and a decontamination procedure proven effective in substantially reducing both the quantity and concentration of lead in housedust, thus substantially reducing blood lead burdens of exposed children.

Acknowledgments

We wish to acknowledge NIEHS Grant ES-01104, "Neurobiology of Environmental Pollutants," Martin Krigman, M.D., and Lester D. Grant, Ph.D., Principal Investigators; USPES Grant HD-03110 to the Child Development Research Institute; MCH Project 916 to the Division for Disorders of Development and Learning, where the children were evaluated and Wake County Public Health Department, Jane Wooten, M.D., Director, where children were also screened. Thanks are also due to the Department of Pediatrics, North Carolina Memorial Hospital, and the Department of Biostatistics for statistical consultation.

References

Baker, E.L., Folland, D.S., Taylor, T.A., Frank, M., Peterson, W., Lovejoy, G., Cox, D., Houseworth, J. and Landrigan, P.J. 1977. Lead poisoning in children of lead workers. New England Journal of Medicine 296:260–261.

Center for Disease Control. Increased lead absorption in children of lead workers—Vermont. Morbidity & Mortality Weekly Report, Feb. 25, 1977.

Dolcourt, J.L., Hamrick, H.J., O'Tuama, L.A., Wooten, J. and Baker, E.L. 1978. Increased lead burden in children of battery workers: Asymptomatic exposure resulting from contaminated work clothing. Pediatrics 62:563–566.

Ediger, R.D. and Coleman, R.L. 1972. Modified Delves Cup atomic absorption procedure for the determination of lead in blood. Atomic Absorption Newsletter 11:33.

Environmental Protection Agency. 1977. Air quality criteria for lead. U.S. Government Printing Office, Washington.

Gleason, M.N., Gosselin, R.E., Hodge, H.C. and Smith, R.R. 1969. Clinical toxicology of commercial products. Williams & Wilkins, Baltimore.

Lepow, M.L., Bruckman, L., Gillette, M., Markowitz, S., Robino, R. and Kapish, J. 1975. Investigations into sources of lead in the environment of urban children. Environmental Research 10:415–426.

Rice, C., Fischbein, A., Lilis, R., Sarkozi, L., Kin, S. and Selikoff, I.J. 1978. Lead contamination in the homes of employees of secondary lead smelters. Environmental Research 15:375–380.

Sayre, J.W., Charney, E., Vostal, J. and Pless, I.B. 1974. House and hand dust as a potential source of childhood lead exposure. American Journal of Diseases of Childhood 127:167–170.

Watson, W.N., Witherall, L.E. and Giguere, G.C. 1978. Increased lead absorption in children of workers in a lead storage battery factory. Journal of Occupational Medicine 20:759–761.

16. Clinical Outpatient Management of Childhood Lead Poisoning

John W. Graef

Introduction

Confronted with an asymptomatic child with evidence of lead toxicity, the clinician has a number of therapeutic choices. His or her dilemma lies in the dearth of data regarding these choices and their outcomes. Even in symptomatic plumbism, whose management Chisolm (1968, 1970, 1974) has pioneered, there exists no controlled study guiding such basic decisions as indications for treatment, duration of treatment or effectiveness of treatment (not in enhancing lead excretion but in preventing or reversing the toxic effects of lead).

In asymptomatic plumbism, the bulk of toxic effects can be measured only in the laboratory and the meaning of these laboratory abnormalities can only be inferred at this time. The landmark study by Needleman et al. (1979) correlating poor school performance with elevated tooth lead indicates that even moderate levels of lead are more toxic than had been demonstrated previously. Nonetheless, while this study encourages the pediatrician to treat such children more aggressively, it does not help him to decide which children to treat, nor when, how, or for how long to treat them.

Other studies, notably those of Sachs et al. (1970), Klein (1977) and Chisolm (1974), describe approaches to management of low level plumbism. However, the outcomes of these studies are measured by a return to normal lab values, not by prevention of long term sequelae. The clinician is left with the knowledge that symptomatic plumbism produces well defined acute and chronic toxic manifestations and that asymptomatic plumbism produces acute and chronic laboratory abnormalities and chronic central nervous system effects. The relation between these latter effects remains to be delineated. The pharmacologic tools for treatment of symptomatic plumbism may not be applicable in the same way to the lower lead level syndrome and at present there exists no well controlled study guiding their use.

In light of this, what follows is a description of the approach used at the Children's Hospital Medical Center in Boston for children with asymptomatic plumbism.

Clinical and Laboratory Evaluation

Blood Level

Table 1 shows some of the criteria used in the clinic to establish the presence of increased lead burden. Blood lead values should be established by means of venous specimens. Although micromethods of blood analysis may be applied to both small and large volumes of blood with comparable precision and accuracy, finger stick (micro) sampling is subject to the contamination which often results in significant error when compared to venous (macro) sampling. Thus, although the finger stick sampling is useful for large scale screening, it is, in our view, too

Table 1. Clinical and laboratory evidence
of lead intoxication and asymptomatic lead burden.

Lead intoxication	Asymptomatic increased lead burden
Clinical	
Anorexia, constipation, irritability, clumsiness, lethargy, behavior changes, hyperactivity (sequela), abdominal pain, vomiting, fever, hepatosplenomegaly, ataxia, convulsions, coma with increased CSF pressure	History of pica Environmental lead source Positive family history Sequelae: fine motor dysfunction, language delay, hyperactivity
Laboratory	
FEP (ZPP) $\geq$ 250 μg/100 ml Microcytic, hypochromic anemia Basophilic erythrocyte stippling Increased urinary coproporphyrin Increased metaphyseal densities on x-ray	Blood lead > 30 μg/100 ml FEP $\geq$ 100 μg/100 ml* Hair lead >100 μg/100 ml in proximal segment 24-hr urinary lead excretion >80–100 μg Lead mobilization test >1 μg/mg EDTA injected/24 hr
Aminoaciduria, glucosuria Prolonged nerve conduction time	Radiopacity in GI tract on x-ray Elevated tooth lead

*FEP $\geq$ 50 μg/100 ml is elevated. However, at moderate elevations, iron deficiency alone may be responsible.

subject to inaccuracy to be used for diagnosis and management. We do not act or form any conclusion until a confirmatory venous lead level has been obtained.

Blood Lead

In some respects, the choice of a blood lead level of 30 μg/dl whole blood as the upper limit of the normal range is arbitrary, although not without foundation. This choice is based on a surprisingly large body of dose-response data in children and adults. These data are summarized in the publications of Zielhuis (1975a, 1975b), the World Health Organization (WHO) (1977) and the United States Environmental Protection Agency (EPA) (1977). The data indicate that the frequency of biochemical evidence of disturbed heme synthesis increases sharply in women and children as blood lead (PbB) rises above 30 μg. The frequency of reduction in hemoglobin seems to increase in children with PbB in the range of 40 to 60 μg. Based on these and other studies, the Center for Disease Control (CDC) (1978) selected a blood lead level of 30 μg as the "action level" in childhood screening programs and chose the erythrocyte protoporphyrin (EP) test (Piomelli et al., 1975) as the primary screening test. Just as there may be children who appear to tolerate blood lead levels about 30 μg without evidence of toxicity (e.g., elevated EP), there are also children with lead levels below 30 μg who may exhibit toxicity at least by laboratory abnormalities (e.g., elevated EP).

Theoretically, it can be argued that the normal blood lead level is zero, in the sense that no essential biological function for lead has ever been found. Nevertheless, lead is one of the constituents of the crust of the earth and measurable amounts of lead are found in the blood of people throughout the world. Indeed, in urban America the mean blood lead level in adults varies from 18 to 23 μg (Blejer, 1976; Smith et al., 1976). When one considers that in vitro inhibition of delta-aminolevulinic acid dehydratase (ALAD) activity in circulating erythrocytes begins at a blood lead level of 10 to 15 μg, it can be argued that most urban Americans exhibit some degree of lead toxicity. The job of the treating physician lies not in determining whether lead toxicity is present, but at what point the potential adverse effects of lead outweigh the risks of treatment.

Erythrocyte Protoporphyrin

According to Piomelli (1975), average normal EP is approximately 20 μg/dl whole blood. The CDC has established ≥50 μg as abnormal for screening purposes (1978). Values as high as 100 μg have often been reported in the presence of iron deficiency and blood lead levels 30 μg/dl whole blood (Stockman et al.). When EP exceeds 100 μg/dl whole blood, some degree of lead effect is likely to be contributing to the elevation. This clearly calls for medical intervention and evaluation of the environment of the child for lead exposure. This interpretation is based on two premises (Goyer and Mahaffey, 1972; Six and Goyer, 1972). The first is that iron deficiency, if present, enhances lead absorption. The second is that iron deficiency tends to occur in children of the same socioeconomic group as those exposed to high lead conditions, irrespective of which condition came first. Lesser elevations of EP in the absence of iron deficiency are indicative of lead toxicity unless proven otherwise.

Hair lead values are included in Table 1, but, in practice, these analyses are difficult to do and the results are subject to error from contamination by atmospheric lead. In any event, hair lead reflects increased excretion of lead due to the high concentration of dithiols in the keratin in hair. Elevated concentrations in the proximal segment of hair are associated with recent but not acute ingestion.

Urinary Lead

Spontaneous 24-hr urinary excretion of lead is elevated in the presence of increased lead burden. Byers and Maloof (1954) pointed out that the concentration of lead in urine varies widely through the day so that results in single samples of urine can be misleading, while total excretion of lead over 24 hr is more reliable. In toilet-trained children and in adults, this measurement is helpful. Greater than 80 to 100 μg/24 hr is indicative of recent increase in exposure.

X-rays

Table 1 includes the presence of radiopacities in the gastrointestinal tract on x-ray. This is listed under asymptomatic increased burden because the mere finding of a radiopacity does not necessarily mean it is lead or, if it is lead, that toxicity has occurred. Nonetheless, because of the high rate of absorption of lead in children and because of the generally high concentration of lead often found in paint chips, a positive abdominal film should be viewed with alarm and diagnostic studies for lead poisoning undertaken immediately. While the absence of a positive film does not rule out pica for paint, the presence of this finding makes one that much more aggressive in pressing for immediate abatement of the source, rapid evaluation and long term surveillance of the child.

X-rays of the long bones, usually knees, are also obtained to look for evidence of metaphyseal sclerosis. Metaphyseal sclerosis is a toxic effect usually requiring maintenance of blood lead levels of about 50 μg% or higher for at least 4 to 6 wk before becoming visible by x-ray. The abnormality is due to the resorption of calcium by osteoclasts and, contrary to common belief, does not represent increased deposition of lead at the metaphyseal plate. Examination of the proximal fibula is most helpful. Because variations in calcium resorption occur normally in 2-yr-olds, lead lines may prove difficult to identify with confidence. However, if the metaphyseal plate of the proximal fibula is dense, the likelihood is that lead and not normal variation is responsible. Because of the time interval required for development of lead lines, their presence is helpful in establishing times of exposure for legal purposes.

Lead Mobilization Test

Among the most helpful tests for increased lead burden is the lead mobilization test. Originally described by Rieders in 1960, this test is based on the premise that if a large dose of chelating agent is administered at one time, the variable controlling the amount of lead excreted over a finite period will be the amount of available or "mobilizable" lead.

Rieders (1960) administered 1 g calcium disodium edetate ($CaNa_2EDTA$) to adults by slow intravenous infusion and collected all urine excreted during the following 24 hr. He proposed that excretion of 1 mg or more of lead in this 24-hr collection (1 μg Pb excreted/1 mg or more CaEDTA administered) constituted evidence of increased body lead burden. Hammond (1973), Teisinger (1971), Teisinger and Srbova (1959) and Chisolm et al. (1975) have confirmed this observation. Statistically, mobilization of 1 μg Pb/1 mg $CaNa_2EDTA$ predicts a mean blood lead concentration of 57 ± 8 μg in children (Chisolm et al., 1976). Because highly statistically significant relationships have been found between the lead mobilization test result and biochemical indicators of deranged heme synthesis (urinary coproporphyrin and delta-aminolevulinic acid output) it has been proposed that the lead mobilization test reflects, at least in part, the potentially toxic or metabolically active portion of the total body lead burden (Chisolm and Harrison, 1956; Selander et al., 1966; Ellis, 1966).

Studies by Foreman (1960) have shown that EDTA is not altered metabolically in the body; rather it is excreted intact exclusively by the kidney. Following intramuscular injection, 80 to 90% of the drug was recovered in the urine within about 4 hr in human adult volunteers. The disappearance of injected PbEDTA in animals follows a somewhat similar temporal pattern. This provides the rationale for the shortened 6- to 8-hr lead mobilization test.

We found that patients defined as having plumbism by other criteria excreted ≥0.5 μg Pb/mg EDTA in 6 to 8 hr. Thus, a child can enter the clinic before 9:00 A.M., void, receive a single intramuscular dose of Versenate (calcium disodium EDTA) and remain in the clinic for a full 6- to 8-hr urine collection. This regimen obviates the need for hospitalization in most cases. Although it is somewhat less reliable than a 24-hr collection, it provides important confirmatory evidence of the presence or absence of a mobilizable pool of lead.

It is important to recognize that a positive lead mobilization test is not synonymous with a diagnosis of lead poisoning. The proven value of the EDTA

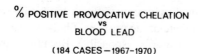

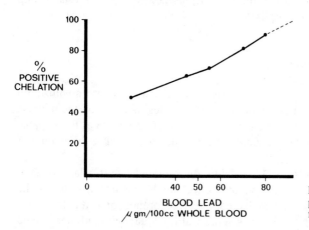

Fig. 1. Percentage of positive provocative chelations as a function of blood lead.

mobilization test is that it demonstrates the effectiveness of EDTA in a given clinical situation. The clinician can utilize this test whenever he questions the need for chelation either in the initial management of a child with lead poisoning or during subsequent follow-up and long term supervision.

Figure 1 depicts per cent positive provocative chelations as a function of blood lead. The data have been compiled from a review of cases at the Children's Hospital Medical Center between 1967 and 1970. Positive lead mobilization tests were obtained in some children with lead levels <40 μg%. Such patients were selected not by screening but by other criteria such as positive x-rays or elevated hair levels. Although free erythrocyte protoporphyrin (FEP) tests have obviated the need for hair leads, x-rays remain useful in selecting cases for provocative chelation.

Table 2 lists some indications for performing the lead mobilization test. Particular attention should be drawn to the last indication, to assess the need for further chelation in the patient already under therapy. In such a case, the lead

Table 2. Indications for lead mobilization test.

1. Venous blood lead $\geq$ 30–60 μg/100 ml and FEP $\geq$ 100 μg/100 ml
2. Venous blood lead $\geq$ 30–60 μg/100 ml and FEP $\geq$ 50–100 μg/100 ml with positive findings on x-rays of abdomen *or* knees
3. To assess need for further chelation in patient under therapy, in whom lead level and FEP may be misleading

level and FEP may be misleading. FEP does not return to normal immediately after chelation, and lead levels are subject to rebound within a few days after chelation. Therefore, absolute figures which are obtained after the end of a 5-day chelation do not accurately reflect the residual lead burden. Only the lead mobilization test can determine whether or not there is a mobilizable pool available for further chelation at the time the test is done.

Therapy

In our clinic, lead poisoned children who are symptomatic, have initial blood lead levels greater than 80 μg% or have renal disease are hospitalized for treatment. Most other children are managed on an outpatient basis if parents can return daily to the clinic. Such management is, of course, complicated by the need for more rapid abatement of the lead hazard than if the child is hospitalized.

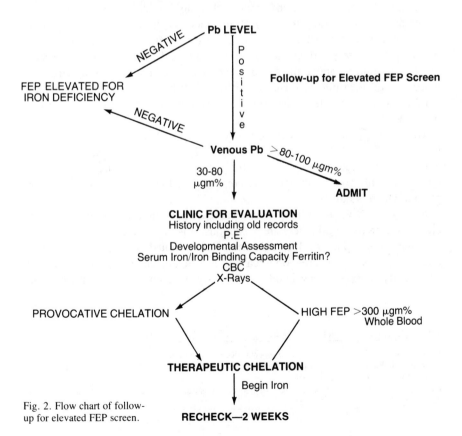

Fig. 2. Flow chart of follow-up for elevated FEP screen.

Nonetheless, the benefits are considerable. They include a reduction in family disruption, the active enlistment of parents in the treatment process with concomitant increased understanding of the disease and its complexities and not least important, a major reduction in the cost of treatment.

Our approach is summarized in the flow sheet on Figure 2. Once confronted with confirmed evidence of toxicity, the clinician must choose appropriate interventions without necessarily knowing whether the final outcome will be altered.

Indications for Chelation

Based on our interpretation of existing studies regarding toxicity of lead, we have established a set of criteria for chelation therapy which are intended as guidelines only (Table 3). In our view, the evidence regarding elevated blood leads is conclusive enough to warrant reducing a blood lead via chelation therapy when it is above 60 μg% for 1 wk or more. While acute ingestions and acute elevations in children do occur, it is our assumption that most children suffer from chronic lowgrade lead ingestion rather than from sudden acute increases. It is also our view that these criteria should apply to all children regardless of age. While it is true that the severest effects are seen in infants and toddlers, we have seen a number of children above the age of 6 who have either suffered long term lead poisoning or intermittent recurrent exposure. When the blood lead of these children is reduced to less than 60 μg%, they seem to show some improvement in behavior.

The second criteria for chelation is a blood lead between 30 and 60 μg/dl together with an FEP greater than or equal to 250 μg/dl. In this case we believe that the FEP is out of the range of simple iron deficiency for most cases and is almost certainly confirmatory of lead poisoning, with the exception of protoporphyria, which is rare.

Finally, we have listed the positive lead mobilization test as an indication for chelation therapy. While there are exceptions, it is our view that once a substantial mobilizable pool of lead has been demonstrated to exist, it should be removed unless there are good reasons not to do so. There are occasions, particularly in very young children who may have undergone multiple chela-

---

Table 3. Indications for chelation therapy.

1. Venous blood lead $\geq$ 60 μg/100 ml on two successive occasions, *or*
2. Venous blood lead $\geq$ 30–60 μg/100 ml and FEP $\geq$ 250 μg/100 ml *or*
3. Positive lead mobilization test

Factors contributing to indications: age, degree of exposure, underlying developmental level, iron deficiency

tions, when a physician may choose to postpone further therapy, recognizing the emotional and physical disruptions which are concomitant to vigorous chelation. Nevertheless, it has also been our experience that when families are enlisted, when careful explanations are given about the need for treatment and when time is spent in comforting and soothing the child, that these considerations, important as they may be, can be kept in perspective in relation to the larger issue of the impact of the continued excessive lead burden on the development of the child.

We have also listed a number of factors which may bear on the decision to treat. These include the age of the child. The younger the child, the more rapidly chelation should be considered and undertaken. Physiologically and developmentally, children under the age of 3 are at greater risk for neurodevelopmental insult from elevated lead levels than are children over the age of 3. We are also more aggressive in treating children with high dose sources of lead, such as paint chips, rather than children with subtle increases in lead burden reflecting mild degrees of exposure.

I feel particularly strongly about treating children whose underlying developmental level is already damaged. After years of custodial care, major efforts are now being made to improve the prognosis for these children and it is difficult to justify allowing them to experience elevated lead levels. Moreover, such children may inhabit a variety of institutions with varying degrees of safety with respect to lead exposure, thus further increasing their risk of toxicity.

Iron Therapy

Perhaps the most important risk factor in determining the need for chelation is the presence of iron or other nutritional deficiency. It is our view that the presence of iron deficiency should make one aggressive about intervention whether or not the intervention initially involves the administration of iron or chelation therapy.

Chelation Protocol

Chisolm has outlined the safe use of chelating agents (1968, 1970, 1974). His contributions have not been improved upon and we have only modified his approach for outpatient use in what is becoming a more widely used form of therapy. CaEDTA is adminstered in single daily intramuscular doses of 50 mg/kg of body weight/day (or 1000 mg/m^2) for 5 successive days. Routine urines are obtained daily and the sediment is examined. Serum BUN, calcium and creatinine are obtained initially and on the fifth day. Parents are counseled to hydrate the child as well as they can during the chelation period. Should signs of renal toxicity appear (initially an increase in white blood cells in the urinary sediment), chelation is discontinued. In more than 800 children treated in this way over the last 5 years in our institution, therapy has had to be discontinued only twice, and in both instances there were unusual circumstances.

The important point is that after 4 to 5 days of therapy, toxicity of CaEDTA increases and the output of mobilizable lead decreases. This increased toxicity coupled with reduced lead diuresis makes the risk-benefit ratio unacceptable after the fifth day, and therapy is then discontinued for a minimum rest period of 48 to 72 hrs. In many cases more lead becomes available for chelation after this period. When the clinician is in doubt as to the need for further chelation, a new lead mobilization test can be performed by collecting urine on the first day of the newly planned 5-day chelation period. Our laboratory can usually determine the urinary lead level within 1 day of receiving the sample, and treatment is discontinued if the urinary excretion appears inadequate to justify further therapy. It should be reiterated that such a test is not foolproof. Ultimately, the decision for therapy must be based on the pattern of lead elevations, the likelihood of further exposure and the response to treatment.

Theoretically, lead bound firmly in bone would seem to leech out into the soft tissues and the blood stream slowly during and after chelation, thereby replenishing the soft tissue compartment and producing the "rebound" blood lead phenomenon. At the same time, the mobilizable pool again increases in size. The soft tissue concentration of lead immediately after chelation has never been measured, and so the dynamics of this process are not well known. After the re-equilibration, however, a new mobilizable pool is available for treatment. With these guidelines in mind, as many chelations as are necessary to reduce the body burden of lead may be performed, providing adequate waiting periods occur between each chelation. New lead mobilization tests can be performed as needed (i.e., 0.5 μg Pb/1 mg EDTA at the start of each chelation). When the values finally become negative, further chelation can be deferred.

An alternative to this approach is that of substituting d-penicillamine in children who are old enough to comply with its prescription for an indefinite period of time. Although not approved by the Food and Drug Administration for use in lead poisoning, d-penicillamine has been shown to be an effective chelating agent in reducing chronic blood lead (Selander, 1966; Selander et al., 1967; Chisolm, 1968; Klein, 1977). We have been able to avoid allergic reactions by instituting initially low doses and doubling them each week until the dose achieved is 20 to 40 mg/kg body weight/24 hr. The child is then maintained for 3 to 6 mos on this dose. In the absence of alternatives, this approach appears to be a realistic way to reduce chronic lead burden. (See Editor's Note, Chapter 18.)

Long Term Management and Follow-Up

We follow all lead poisoned children until they are in school and, occasionally, longer. Follow-up includes periodic laboratory assessment (i.e., lead, FEP and complete blood count) and social and neuropsychological assessments.

Specifically, lead and FEP are followed monthly until they either return to normal or until further intervention is undertaken. Once the values are normal, we usually ask the family to return at increasing intervals of 3 mos, 6 mos and 1 yr. Our staff, particularly social services, is available when the family needs assistance. At a mutually convenient time after the fourth birthday of the child or earlier, if indicated, a neuropsychological assessment is obtained to identify any deficits as early as possible. The lead clinic staff then participates in school initiated assessments and in the formulation of education plans.

Summary

Tables 1-3 summarize our approach to outpatient management. The goal of management is to reduce safely the body burden of lead to acceptable levels as quickly as possible. As more data become available regarding the use of iron and other nutrients including zinc, ascorbic acid and citrate, the need for chelation may be reduced. Nevertheless, the clinician should familiarize himself with chelation therapy and not hesitate to use it as needed. Finally, long term follow-up is essential to adequate management both to avoid recurrence and to assist the child in overcoming any developmental deficits which may have resulted from his or her disease.

References

Baloh, R.W. 1974. Laboratory diagnosis of increased lead absorption. Arch Environ Health 28:198–207.

Blejer, H. 1976. Inorganic lead: Biological indices of absorption—biological threshold limit values. In: Health Effects of Occupational Lead and Arsenic Exposure. Carnow, B., Ed. US DHEW. Chicago. 165–178.

Braitman, R. 1978. Letter to the Editor. Marked elevation of FEP with iron deficiency anemia. J Pediatr 93:155–156.

Byers, R.K. and Maloof, C.C. 1954. Edathmil calcium-disodium (versenate) in treatment of lead poisoning in children. Amer J Dis Child 87:559.

Center for Disease Control. 1978. Preventing Lead Poisoning in Young Children. U.S. DHEW. Public Health Service.

Chisolm, J.J. Jr. 1970. Treatment of acute lead intoxication: Choice of chelating agents and supportive therapy measures. Clin Toxicol 3:527–570.

Chisolm, J.J. Jr. 1974. Chelation therapy in children with subclinical plumbism. Pediatrics 53:441–443.

Chisolm, J.J. Jr., Barrett, M.D. and Harrison, M.V. 1975. Indicators of internal dose of lead in relation to derangement in heme synthesis. Johns Hopkins Med J 173:6–12.

Chisolm, J.J. Jr. and Harrison, H.E. 1956. Quantitative urinary coproporphyrin excretion and its relation to edathamil calcium disodium administration in children with acute lead intoxication, J Clin Invest 35:1131–1138.

Ellis, R.W. 1966. Urinary screening tests to detect excessive lead absorption, Br J Ind Med 23:263–281.

Environmental Protection Agency. Air Quality Criteria for Lead. EPA 600/8-77-017, December, 1977.

Goyer, R. and Mahaffey, K. 1972. Susceptibility to lead toxicity. Environ Health Perspect 4:73–80.

Hammond, P.B. 1973. The relationship between inhibition of delta-aminolevulinic acid dehydratase by lead and lead mobilization by ethylenediamine tetraacetate (EDTA). Toxicol Appl Pharm 26:466–475.

Klein, R. 1977. Lead poisoning. In Advances in Pediatrics. Barness, L.A., Ed. Year Book Medical Publishers, Chicago. 111–115.

Needleman, H.L., Gunnoe, C., Leviton, A., Reed, R., Peresie, H., Maher, C. and Barrett, P. 1979. Deficits in psychologic and classroom performance of children with elevated dentine lead levels. NEJM 300:689–695.

Piomelli, S., Davidow, B. and Guinee, V.F. 1973. The FEP (free erythrocyte porphyrins) test: A screening micromethod for lead poisoning. Pediatrics 51:254.

Piomelli, S. et al. 1975. J Clin Invest 56:1519.

Rabinowitz, M.B., Wetherill, G.W. and Kopple, J.D. 1976. Kinetic analysis of lead metabolism in healthy humans. J Clin Invest 58:260–270.

Rieders, F. 1960. Current concepts in the therapy of lead poisoning. In Metal Binding in Medicine. Sever, H.J., Ed. J.B. Lippincott, Philadelphia. 143–455.

Sachs, H.K. et al. 1970. Ambulatory treatment of lead poisoning. Report of 1,155 cases. Pediatrics 46:389.

Saritain, P., Whitaker, J. and Martin, J. 1964. The absence of lead lines in bones of children with early lead poisoning. Amer J Roentgen 91.

Selander, S. 1967. Treatment of lead poisoning. A comparison between the effects of sodium calcium-edatate and penicillamine administered orally and intravenously. Brit J Indust Med 24:272–282.

Selander, S., Cramer, K. and Hallberg, L. 1966. Studies in lead poisoning. Oral therapy with penicillamine: Relationship between lead in blood and other laboratory tests. Brit J Indust Med 23:282–290.

Six, K.M. and Goyer, R.A. 1972. The influence of iron deficiency on tissue content and toxicity of ingested lead in the rat. J Lab Clin Med 79:128–136.

Smith, T.J., Temple, A.R. and Reading, J.C. 1976. Cadmium lead and copper blood levels in normal children. Clin Toxicol 9:75–87.

Stockman, J.A. III, Weiner, L.S., Simon, G.E., Stuart, M.J. and Oski, F.A. 1975. The measurement of free erythrocyte prophyrin (FEP) as a simple means of distinguishing iron deficiency from beta-thalassemia trait in subjects with microcytosis. J Lab Clin Med 35:113–119.

Teisinger, J. 1971. Biochemical responses to provocative chelation by edetate disodium calcium. Arch Environ Health 23:280–283.

Teisinger, J. and Srbova, J. 1959. The value of mobilization of lead by calcium ethylene-diamine-tetra-acetate in the diagnosis of lead poisoning. Brit J Indust Med 16:148–152.

World Health Organization (WHO). Lead III. Geneva.

Zielhuis, R.L. 1975a. Dose-response relationships for inorganic lead. I. Biochemical and haematological responses. Int Arch Occup Health 35:1–18.

Zielhuis, R.L. 1975b. Dose-response relationships for inorganic lead. II. Subjective and functional responses-chronic sequelae-no-response levels. Int Arch Occup Health 35:19–35.

17. Role of the Pediatric Intermediate Care Facility in the Treatment of Children with Lead Poisoning

Paul Burgan

When presented with a child whose body content of lead is toxic or potentially toxic, the primary goal is to reduce the lead burden. This can be done either by decreasing the rate by which lead is entering the body or by increasing the rate at which it is leaving the body. For fastest results, both means can be utilized. This reduction in lead burden should be accomplished with as little physical and emotional disturbance as possible.

Other goals in treating these children with lead poisoning are to prevent recurrences and to look for signs of brain damage so that appropriate treatment may be instituted and proper educational placement made.

The most common method of treatment is to admit the child to an acute care hospital for a period of parenteral chelation therapy, usually with calcium disodium edetate (CaEDTA). The child is then seen as an outpatient and, if the lead level increases again, is retreated. Dr. Graef describes an outpatient approach to treatment (Chapter 16).

Another method of treatment utilizes the services available at a pediatric intermediate care facility. Although only 18 such facilities exist in the United States, the intermediate care concept may be applicable even where such a facility is not available.

Mt. Washington Pediatric Hospital, in Baltimore, Maryland, is a 62-bed intermediary and long term care hosnital. Children whose medical condition is stable enough that they do not require the services of an acute care hospital yet have requirements that cannot be met at home are admitted until further improvement in their status or the family's ability to provide care allows them to return home. The hospital provides extensive physical therapy, psychology, speech, social work and educational services in addition to medical and nursing services. Children are admitted directly from home or are transferred from other hospitals. The advantages of this type of hospital are the ability to focus on the long term social, emotional and educational needs of children and the ability to provide these services at about half the per diem cost of an acute care facility.

In 1979, 77 children with increased lead were admitted to Mt. Washington Pediatric Hospital. This represents about 20% of all children with identified Class 3 or Class 4 lead levels in Baltimore during that period. About 75% of the children admitted to Mt. Washington Pediatric Hospital were detected initially by the Baltimore City Health Department screening program and by Dr. Julian Chisolm. The remainder were detected by a variety of health maintenance organizations and other primary care providers. About 20% of the admissions were treated elsewhere prior to coming to Mt. Washington Pediatric Hospital, in most cases because a bed was not immediately available and their condition required immediate chelation therapy. The blood leads of the children prior to admission ranged from 38 to 81 μg/dl. Free erythrocyte protoporphyrin (FEP) ranged from 300 to 1534 μg/dl of erythrocytes (RBC). For about 10% of the children this was the second time that treatment for increased lead was required.

Upon admission to Mt. Washington, these children were treated with CaEDTA for 5 days, if this had not already been done. They were then placed on daily oral d-penicillamine. D-penicillamine was continued for as long as there was evidence of significant lead burden. The children were placed on low fat diets supplemented with iron and mineral preparations. Urinalysis, hematological studies to assess anemia and blood chemistries to measure hepatic and renal function were routinely obtained. Blood counts (CBC) were obtained at weekly intervals to measure absolute neutrophil count. While on penicillamine, 10% of children will show a fall in the absolute neutrophil count to less than 1500, which is considered an adverse drug reaction necessitating discontinuation of d-penicillamine. When the neutrophil count rose quickly (i.e., in 7 to 10 days), a second trial of oral d-penicillamine was given, usually at a lower dose. For the small number of children who showed repeated decreases in their neutrophil count, d-penicillamine was discontinued entirely.

(Editors' Note: A complete blood count including differential white blood cell count should be done weekly during the first month of d-penicillamine therapy and at least monthly thereafter while the patient is receiving the drug. We are aware of instances in which an absolute neutrophil count of 500 or less was found when the child's blood was first tested after a few weeks of d-penicillamine therapy. Fortunately, even in these cases the reaction was reversible upon stopping the drug.)

The average length of stay of the children was 63 days with a range of 20 to 104 days. These figures do not include patients who were readmitted for a repeat course of CaEDTA. (This was done if there had been a previous adverse response to d-penicillamine.) At the time of discharge blood leads ranged from 13 to 29 μg/dl, and FEP ranged from 83 to 273 μg/dl RBC. Usually patients are discharged when FEP is about 150 μg/dl RBC. Children discharged with higher levels are those whose home has been cleared of lead hazards and whose family is felt to be reliable. In this group of patients, the child with a FEP of 83 μg/dl RBC had been admitted twice before and had a very disorganized family with whom we were trying to work as long as possible to reduce the risk of another occurrence. After discharge, all children continued to be followed for evidence of recurrence, generally at the referring facility.

During hospitalization of a child at the Mt. Washington Pediatric Hospital, the Baltimore City Health Department inspects the home for the presence of lead. After removal of lead the home is reinspected to insure that lead hazards have been abated in compliance with local ordinances. Unfortunately, this process may be lengthy.

Our social work staff works intensively with the family to deal with the stresses produced by the long hospitalization and to address changes which can be made in the family structure. The child life and education staff provides pre-school, school and recreational programs to help minimize the negative effects of hospitalization. The nursing staff provides emotional as well as physical support for these children. The nursing and child life staffs use behavioral modification techniques to reduce pica and mouthing behavior. Physical therapy and psycho-logical hearing and speech evaluations are routinely done on all children, and therapy is instituted where appropriate. An educational program is used to teach the family about lead, good nutrition and the basics of good child-rearing practices.

Reports accumulate of the adverse effects of lead levels previously thought to be safe. Until techniques to determine when the brain is at risk are developed, earlier and more aggressive treatment seems indicated. To provide such treatment with least disturbance to the child and least cost to the community requires the availability of a variety of options to meet individual case needs. The use of an intermediate care facility is one such option.

Editors' Historical Note

In the early 1950's, J.J. Chisolm, Jr., reviewed cases of acute childhood lead poisoning at The Johns Hopkins Hospital and the Baltimore City Hospitals where the majority of children with lead poisoning in the city then received their care.

Most of the children admitted to the inpatient service had acute encephalopathy. During the decade prior to 1953, most of the children were treated with chelation therapy and upon subsidence of symptoms were discharged home, usually within a few weeks. A review revealed that recurrences of acute encephalopathy were frequent and that re-exposure to flaking lead paint in the home and recurrence of symptomatic lead poisoning increased the prevalence of severe brain damage among survivors to virtually 100% (Chisolm and Harrison, 1956). The review also revealed that a number of children admitted for acute encephalopathy had had elevated blood lead concentrations a few weeks or months prior to their admission for acute encephalopathy. Because they were asymptomatic, they were sent home only to return, severely ill, shortly thereafter. These facts made it evident that brief courses of chelation therapy were of limited benefit in the long term management of these children unless some means could be found to separate them promptly from their source of lead, which was flaking lead paint in virtually all cases. It also became evident that pediatric intervention would have to take place in the early asymptomatic stage if strides in the prevention of severe lead poisoning and its sequellae were to be made. In 1951, the City of Baltimore passed the first local ordinance to prohibit the use of lead paint on dwelling interiors. This was incorporated in the Hygiene of Housing Code in 1954 and read in part as follows: "No paint shall be used for interior painting on any dwelling, dwelling unit, rooming house or rooming unit unless the paint is free from any lead pigment." Under this ordinance, the Baltimore City Health Department used its powers to enforce the removal of lead pigment paint in the homes of children with either symptomatic plumbism or asymptomatic increased lead absorption (i.e., PbB >60 μg, which was then considered the upper limit of normal in children). However, then as now, abatement of lead hazards within the home took a very long time, often from 1 to 3 mos or longer. Our experience showed that recurrences of lead encephalopathy could indeed occur within this short time. Some safe intermediate place between the acute care hospital and home was needed if the grim prognosis in such cases was to be improved.

In August of 1953, Dr. Chisolm approached the staff of the Happy Hills Hospital, or Mt. Washington Pediatric Hospital as it is called today, about transferring children from the major acute pediatric hospitals to Happy Hills Hospital for further therapy after the acute stage of clinical illness. The vast majority of patients at Happy Hills at that time were school-aged children convalescing from acute rheumatic fever. Inasmuch as rheumatic fever was declining, the timing of this request was propitious, for the institution was receptive to the idea of new types of patients. The staff agreed and the first patient, a 20-mo-old boy, was transferred from The Johns Hopkins Hospital to Happy Hills in August, 1953. This patient was somewhat rambunctious, which disturbed the nursing staff, who for many years had been used to handling well-behaved older children. Dr. Chisolm carefully selected the next patient for good behavior, a little girl who endeared herself to the staff. Since that time, Mt.

Washington Pediatric Hospital has served as a vital community resource in the management of children with chronic plumbism, both asymptomatic and symptomatic. Indeed, the availability of this facility has enabled pediatricians in Baltimore to undertake a preventive approach to lead toxicity. Originally, asymptomatic children, often siblings or housemates of an index case, were admitted to Mt. Washington Pediatric Hospital if their blood lead concentration exceeded 60 μg/dl whole blood. As noted by Dr. Burgan, admitting criteria permit the admission of children at an even earlier stage of increased lead absorption today. Discharge from this institution from the very beginning has been keyed to finding safe housing for the child and his family. This could be achieved through either abatement of the lead hazards in the home of the child according to current ordinances or relocation of the family into public housing, which in Baltimore has been "lead free" since the inception of the public housing program in 1938. From the first, the use of lead paints in public housing has been prohibited. The availability of the Mt. Washington Pediatric Hospital coupled with the aggressive persistence of the Bureau of Industrial Hygiene of the Baltimore City Health Department and the comprehensive plan outlined by Burgan played a major role in improving the prognosis of childhood lead poisoning in Baltimore in the 1950's and 1960's. The institution continues to provide this and other vitally important community services today, although it is no longer the only intermediate care facility in the United States caring for children with plumbism, as it was in earlier years.

References

Chisolm, J.J. Jr. and Harrison, H.E. 1956. The Exposure of Children to Lead. Pediatrics 18:943.

18. Management of Increased Lead Absorption— Illustrative Cases

J. Julian Chisolm, Jr.

A general overview of therapy has been presented by Dr. Graef (Chapter 16) and an overview of the role of the intermediate care facility has been presented by Dr. Burgan (Chapter 17). I would like now to move from the general to the particular, using individual case histories from our clinic to illustrate several of the varied problems that the treating physician may encounter in outpatient management. For the past eight years, the Lead Clinic at the John F. Kennedy Institute has served as a referral center for the Baltimore metropolitan area. Cases are referred from primary care facilities where initial screening is done. The clinic has 350 to 400 active cases at any one time. Emphasis is placed upon a detailed environmental history. A most important and possibly unique feature is the clinic laboratory, where blood lead (PbB) and free erythrocyte protoporphyrin (FEP) tests are done while the patient waits; this greatly facilitates immediate decisions regarding management. Other tests described by Dr. Graef (Chapter 16) are used on a selective basis.

Before proceeding to the presentation of cases, I would like to stress some points in the rationale of the approach used in this clinic. While it is true that chelation therapy has never been evaluated, as many drugs are, through a controlled prospective study to compare outcome in treated and untreated children with either symptomatic plumbism or asymptomatic increased lead absorption, it is doubtful that such a study will ever be done, given the ethical constraints now applied to research in children. On the other hand, the acute toxic effects of lead on the kidney and bone marrow are quickly reversed during chelation therapy. In addition, at least three retrospective clinical reports indicate that shortening of the period of increased soft tissue lead concentrations during the preschool years (as indicated by blood lead concentrations elevated above the 40 to 50 μg range) may improve outcome as measured by psychometric tests of cognitive function when school age is reached (Rummo, 1977; Pueschel et al., 1972; Albert et al., 1974). To reduce the duration of increased lead absorption, we place major emphasis on reduction of exposure, inasmuch as brief periods of chelation therapy may be of little or no avail if the child continues to live under the same high exposure conditions. Exposure may be reduced not only through the removal of scaling leaded paint in and about the child's residence, but also through reduction in exposure to lead-containing dust. The data presented by Charney (Chapter 8), Milar and Mushak (Chapter 15) and Sobolesky (Chapter 14) emphasize the importance of reducing exposure to fine particulate lead through suppression of dust in the home and play areas.

The available dose-response data in humans show that the risk of long lasting adverse effects of lead rises sharply as PbB rises above the 50 μg level (Rummo, 1977; WHO, 1977). I have generally limited chelation therapy to patients with venous PbB $\geqslant$50 μg. Our recent studies show that the FEP test (Piomelli et al., 1973; Chisolm and Brown, 1975) is not predictive of therapeutic response to calcium disodium edetate (CaEDTA) in children (Chisolm et al., 1979). While the FEP test is useful in overall evaluation of risk and in long term responses to management, it has only a very limited role in the initial selection of patients for chelation therapy. Chelation therapy is given in hospital, be it a 3- to 5-day course of intramuscular CaEDTA or an initial 5-day course of CaEDTA (1000 mg/m^2/day) followed by oral d-penicillamine (not exceeding 500 mg/m^2/day). Outpatient chelation therapy is given only if the following two conditions are met: 1) the child resides in a low lead environment (i.e., modern or "lead-free" public housing) and 2) the parents are able to comply with proper administration of oral d-penicillamine and frequent visits to the clinic for adequate monitoring of drug therapy. Practically speaking, when these two conditions are met, chelation therapy is often not needed. Furthermore, owing to the lack of such "safe" housing in Baltimore, this option is not available for the vast majority of our patients. We do not give chelation therapy on an outpatient basis to children residing in old housing, even if lead hazards have been abated according to current local ordinances, which require removal of lead pigment paints only up to the 4-ft level. Scaling paint above this level is not necessarily removed. Screening data in children in older housing in the decaying parts of the city have shown a remarkably constant and elevated blood lead level (mean PbB = 38 to 40 μg) for at least the past 30 years (Kaplan and McDonald, 1942; Bradley et al., 1956; Chisolm et al., 1976). Follow-up data from the Kennedy Institute Lead Clinic currently show that children returned to abated old housing reach and maintain this same average PbB, namely, 40 μg, usually within 3 months (J.J. Chisolm, Jr., unpublished data). This is indicative of persistent low level increased lead exposure. Experimental data strongly suggest that administration of chelating agents in the presence of over-exposure to lead may be not only ineffectual but

Table 1.   Influence of intraperitoneal administration of calcium disodium ethylenediamine-tetraacetate (EDTA) and 2,3-dimercaptopropanol (BAL) in equimolar concentration (0.2 mmol/kg*) on absorption, whole-body retention and total Urinary excretion of single oral dose of Pb^{203} given with stable lead (50 mg/kg) acetate[†] (Jugo et al., 1975).

Group	Whole-body Retention	Total Urinary Excretion	Absorption[‡]
Control (N = 18)	1.05 ± 0.14	0.13 ± 0.02	1.19 ± 0.15
CaEDTA (N = 20)	1.47 ± 0.24	1.54 ± 0.29	3.01 ± 0.50
BAL (N = 20)	1.60 ± 0.28	1.45 ± 0.24	3.05 ± 0.49

*This is 0.2 mmol/kg = 67.5 mg CaEDTA/kg and 22.5 mg BAL/kg.
[†]The results are expressed as a percentage of dose (mean ± SEM) 144 hr after administration of lead and chelating agent.
[‡]Absorption was calculated by adding total urinary excretion to whole body retention.

also potentially hazardous in that it can actually increase the body lead burden if lead and a chelating agent are present in the gut simultaneously. Reiders (1954) gave lead and CaEDTA orally to rabbits and found that fecal lead excretion was reduced and urinary lead excretion was increased, but total lead excretion remained unaltered. On the basis of his and other studies, oral administration of CaEDTA had been strongly condemned since the early 1950's. The more recent studies of Jugo et al. (1975) are summarized in Tables 1 and 2. Even when CaEDTA is given parenterally and lead orally, absorption of lead from the gut is increased and one-half of the absorbed dose is retained (Table 1). The portion retained is marginally greater than the portion retained by controls which received lead in a highly absorbable chemical form such as lead acetate. In order to simulate the presence of lead and chelating agent together in the gut, Jugo et al. (1975) also administered various metal chelates orally. These experiments (Table 2) confirmed those of Reiders (1954) for lead-EDTA and showed, in addition, that retention of lead is substantially increased when oral lead-penicillamine is given. These data have led me to be extremely cautious regarding outpatient chelation therapy. Even in hospital, d-penicillamine is given on an empty stomach, usually in the early morning at least two hours before breakfast.

Table 2.   Absorption, whole-body retention and total urinary excretion of Pb^{203} 144 hr after a single oral dose of some lead chelates to rats* (Jugo et al., 1975).

	Whole-body Retention	Total Urinary Excretion	Absorption[†]
Control (Pb-acetate) (N = 8)	0.70 ± 0.15	0.31 ± 0.05	1.01 ± 0.20
Pb-EDTA (N = 10)	0.43 ± 0.04	1.39 ± 0.13	1.82 ± 0.14
Pb-penicillamine (N = 7)	1.87 ± 0.19	1.22 ± 0.10	3.09 ± 0.28
Pb-BAL (N = 10)	3.39 ± 0.44	6.62 ± 0.96	9.94 ± 1.31

*Dose of stable lead was 0.5 mg/kg and doses of chelating agents were 0.2 mmol/kg. The results are expressed as a percentage of dose (mean ± SEM).
[†]Absorption was calculated by adding total urinary excretion to whole-body retention.

Illustrative Cases

Highly Elevated FEP with Normal or Moderately Elevated PbB

A not uncommon problem is presented by the child in whom the elevation in FEP seems disproportionately high in comparison with PbB. Ordinarily, this combination indicates that the child has iron deficiency, either latent or manifest, and if PbB ⩾ 30, increased lead absorption. We often encounter children with PbB ⩾ 50 μg and iron deficiency anemia (hemoglobin < 11gm %) with FEP in the range of 1,000 to 3,000 μg/dl erythrocytes. Such cases receive not only chelation therapy for lead but also vigorous oral iron therapy. The vexing problem arises when hematocrit falls within the normal range, PbB is in the 30 to 49 μg range and FEP is highly elevated. This combination would upgrade the child's status from Class II to Class IV according to current CDC risk classification (Center for Disease Control, 1978). How such a child is handled in this clinic is illustrated by the following case.

Case 1. Laboratory data at the initial clinic visit in a 20-mo-old toddler showed the following: FEP = 925 μg/dl erythrocytes, PbB = 47 μg and Hct = 35%. He resided in a dilapidated old house. History indicated deficient dietary intake of iron and subsequent laboratory tests showed latent iron deficiency, although hemoglobin (11 gm %) was normal. These data and his course are shown in Figure 1. He was treated with oral iron (5 mg Fe/kg/day). During the first 7 wk, FEP decreased and hematocrit increased while PbB remained unchanged. At this point, the family moved to "lead-free" public housing on the periphery of the city, whereupon, FEP continued to decrease and PbB began to decrease, eventually reaching the normal range after approximately 6 mos.

This case illustrates the degree to which moderately increased lead absorption and latent iron deficiency may elevate FEP. Since chelatable lead is related to PbB and not to FEP (Chisolm et al., 1976; Chisolm et al., 1979), medicinal iron but not chelation therapy is used in cases such as this when PbB <50 μg.

Other less common disproportionate FEP-PbB pairs may be difficult to interpret. Spectrophotofluorometric studies are done when FEP is disproportionately elevated in order to determine whether zinc protoporphyrin or protoporphyrin IX or a mixture of the two are present (Chisolm and Brown, 1979). In sickle cell disease, 20 to 50% of the total FEP (zinc protoporphyrin plus protoporphyrin IX) may be protoporphyrin IX. The presence of protoporphyrin IX appears to be related to the presence of increased numbers of very immature erythrocytes in the circulating blood. Even so, we are still left with a small number of cases in which FEP, due almost exclusively to zinc protoporphyrin, is greatly elevated (500 to 1,000 μg/dl erythrocytes), but PbB < 30 μg. Chelatable lead is not increased. No confirmatory evidence of iron deficiency is obtained, no hemoglobinopathy is found and there is no evidence of a chronic hemolytic process (i.e., normal haptoglobin and hemopexin). These cases have been tentatively classified as "elevated FEP, etiology undetermined." In a few such cases follow-up over several years has shown a slow decline in FEP.

Chelation Therapy under "Safe" Housing Conditions

Sometimes parental resources and motivation combine favorably with transfer to safe modern housing. This, in turn, can permit the extended use of oral d-penicillamine on an outpatient basis as illustrated by the following case.

Case 2. This toddler was first screened at a primary care clinic at 20 mos of age on June 20. Subsequently, the laboratory reported the following: PbB = 72 μg; FEP = 334 μg/dl erythrocytes. She was referred to our clinic, arriving 4 wk later when PbB = 81 μg and FEP = 433 μg. She was immediately admitted to the Pediatric Clinical Research Unit of the Johns Hopkins Hospital for further evaluation and chelation therapy. Her course over the next 30 mo, as depicted by serial PbB and FEP data, is summarized in Figure 2. On admission, her mother reported that she had been irritable and vomited three or four times during the preceding fortnight; however, no symptoms were observed by the nursing staff during her hospitalization. Psychometric evaluation revealed normal developmental progress and cognitive function at the time. Hospitalization terminated her overexposure and by the fourth day in the hospital, just prior to starting CaEDTA, PbB had decreased spontaneously from 81 to 69 μg, while FEP continued to increase, reaching its peak on the fourteenth hospital day. Just prior to therapy, spontaneous urinary lead output was 22 μg Pb/day and urinary δ-aminolevulinic acid (ALAU) was 4.11 mg/m^2/day (normal, 1.13 ± 0.34 mg/m^2/day). Chelatable lead, as measured on the first day of CaEDTA therapy, was 674 μg Pb/day or 1.35 μg Pb/1 mg CaEDTA administered. CaEDTA was discontinued after 5 days and oral d-penicillamine was begun and tolerated well for the next 4 mos, as indicated by the solid segments of the lines in Figure 2. Little progress was being made in the abatement of the lead hazards in her dilapidated home; however, the child was discharged to the paternal grandmother, who lived in public housing. Some weeks later the parents did find an apartment in a new housing development (less than 15 yr old) on the periphery of the city and near the mother's place of employment. This housing development also had day care facilities for working mothers. The child was in "safe" housing and was discharged on d-penicillamine, which was continued for an additional 3.5 mos.

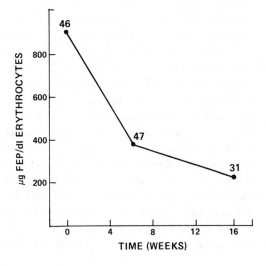

Fig. 1. Combined influence of iron deficiency and increased lead absorption on erythrocyte protoporphyrin (FEP). Line connecting points shows trend in FEP during oral iron therapy while numbers adjacent to points show PbB values. Additional data (serum iron = 21 μg/dl; TIBC = 544 μg/dl; percent saturation = 3.9%; hematocrit = 35%) provide substantiating evidence of iron deficiency while PbB indicates moderate increase in lead absorption initially (Chisolm and Barltrop, 1979).

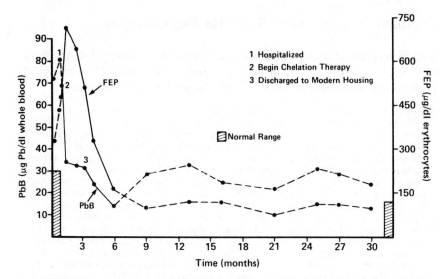

Fig. 2. Inpatient and outpatient chelation therapy under "safe" housing conditions. Lines show trends in blood lead (PbB) and "free" erythrocyte protoporphyrin (FEP) as indicated in the figure. Solid segments of the lines indicate the period during which chelation therapy was given, while dashed segments of the lines indicate periods when patient was not receiving chelation therapy. Numbers in circles show points at which patient was hospitalized (1), begun on chelation therapy (2) and discharged to modern housing (3). Bars adjacent to the scales for PbB and FEP indicate normal ranges for these measurements.

This case illustrates several points. The delay between initial screening and arrival at the referral clinic was unduly long, perhaps made so by the total time taken in transport of the sample to a central laboratory, actual analysis and transmittal of the report to the screening facility. Additional time was needed to locate the mother due to the fact that she worked, had no telephone and left the child with a babysitter, whose address was not known to the primary screening facility. The delayed response in FEP is also notable; indeed, it is usual for FEP to continue rising or remain stable for 2 to 3 wk after the institution of chelation therapy before it begins to decrease. Upon stopping d-penicillamine, PbB rebounded but FEP, having fallen to approximately 150 μg/dl erythrocytes, continued to decrease. This, too, is usual when chelation therapy is stopped in patients at a time when they are not over-exposed to lead. Presumably, this combination reflects transitory internal redistribution of lead. In patients who are unduly re-exposed after chelation therapy, both PbB and FEP tend to rise concurrently, which in turn indicates that a second course of chelation therapy should receive consideration. This particular child has remained in modern housing during the subsequent 24 mos of follow-up off d-penicillamine. PbB has undulated seasonally between 22 and 31 μg with peaks during the summer and valleys during the winter months. At 4 yr of age and 21 mos after the initial detection, psychometric evaluation shows normal development and average intelligence. Only about 10% of patients attending our clinic are able to secure safe housing. More recent experience suggests that chelation therapy is probably unnecessary in most young children who move to "safe" housing immediately after inpatient treatment. Many such children show spontaneous improvement upon reduction in environmental exposure, as illustrated by Case 5. If such cases show rebound in PbB, they may be treated alternatively by 3- to 5-day courses of CaEDTA.

Mobility of Families and Long-term Management

Families in rental property in high risk urban areas tend to move frequently which both complicates long term follow-up and makes it not only difficult but also essential. They may move from old housing in good condition to dilapidated old houses and vice versa. The course of one such case, summarized in Figure 3, typifies this problem.

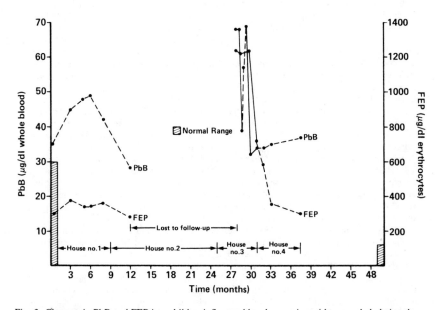

Fig. 3. Changes in PbB and FEP in a child as influenced by changes in residence and chelation therapy in hospital. Bars adjacent to the scales for PbB and FEP indicate normal ranges for these measurements. Trends in PbB and FEP are as indicated in figure. Changes in residence are indicated as house numbers 1, 2, 3 and 4. The period during which the child was lost to follow-up is also indicated in the figure.

Case 3. This child has been followed for 3 yr and is being followed because the issue of over-exposure is not as yet resolved. She was 32 mos of age when first seen at the Kennedy Institute Lead Clinic and 68 mos of age at the most recent visit. During this time she has lived in four different residences as noted in Figure 3. When first seen, the child's blood lead concentration was slightly elevated and steadily increased over the next 6 mos. Her mother reported that the child had pica for paint, paper and dirt and that she constantly sucked her thumb. Areas of flaking paint were reported by the mother. Inspection by the Health Department indicated the presence of lead hazards, not only in the child's primary residence, but also in her aunt's house across the street, where she spent a considerable amount of time. At the first visit the patient was one of three children less than 7 yr of age and the mother was in the third trimester of pregnancy. During the period in which the child's blood lead concentration increased over the ensuing 6 mos abatement of lead hazards was being carried out spasmodically in her own home and in her aunt's home across the street. Although the child was out of the home during the actual burning and sanding of paint, she spent each night at home. The rise in blood lead concentration was attributed to her presence in the home during this process. At 9-mos follow-up, PbB had begun to decrease but the mother moved at this time to another old but recently thoroughly renovated home with new woodwork and panelling throughout. Three months after this move, the child's blood lead concentration had decreased to 28 μg Pb, a value within the normal range. The mother was advised of this improvement but told to continue oral iron medication because of incompletely treated associated iron deficiency. However, the mother failed to keep follow-up appointments for the next 16 mos. The case was referred to the Health Department for tracing and for follow-up; however, the child did not return for 16 mos, nor is any record available to indicate that she was tested elsewhere.

She was next seen at 60 mos of age at a well-baby clinic and referred back to the Kennedy Institute where a blood lead concentration of 67 μg % and a highly elevated FEP (1243 μg/dl erythrocytes) were found and the child was immediately admitted to the Clinic Research Unit for evaluation and treatment. The mother reported that the child had shown increased irritability during the preceding fortnight; however, no other symptoms were reported which would be compatible with early clinical plumbism. Three months prior to this admission, the mother moved to House Number 3 (Figure 3), which she said was in a severe state of dilapidation with much chipping and flaking paint. This was confirmed by Health Department inspection. Lead was reported in the chipping paint throughout the house. Additional laboratory data revealed no evidence of hemoglobinopathy or iron deficiency. Psychometric testing showed a borderline low general cognitive index on the McCarthy Scales (IQ = 78). Prior to treatment, spontaneous urinary lead output was 47 μg/24 hr., ALAU was 7.03 mg/m^2/24 hr. and the first day's urinary lead output during CaEDTA was 1.24 μg Pb excreted/1 mg CaEDTA administered. Long bone x-rays were positive for metaphyseal sclerosis ("lead lines"). No symptoms were observed in hospital by the nursing staff. There was no change in PbB during the three days prior to CaEDTA, suggestive of a rather long standing increase in lead absorption. The mother had obtained information from the City Housing Department, on the basis of her long standing application, that she would have a totally renovated subsidized home within 6 wk. In the meantime, the mother stated that she would have the child stay permanently with an aunt in a rehabilitated housing unit until her own home was available. She was, therefore, discharged to be followed at fortnightly intervals until the housing situation was settled. During the month following discharge, blood lead concentration rose from 39 to 69 μg, while FEP remained essentially unchanged at 1200 to 1250 μg/dl erythrocytes. The child was readmitted for study. Again, urinary ALA and lead data revealed the same changes found at the first admission. These data were strongly suggestive of re-exposure. Following the initial phase of treatment, the child was transferred to Mt. Washington Pediatric Hospital for continuation of therapy with d-penicillamine. After a month's hospitalization, the mother signed the child out, although she had not, as yet, secured "safe" housing. This time she agreed to allow the child and her similarly affected sister to live with the grandmother, who had secured completely renovated housing in an old housing area of the city. Inspection of this home has revealed no hazardous flaking lead-containing paints. PbB seems to be stabilizing at 35 to 40 μg. This, in our experience, is average for young children living in the older areas of the city, even in houses which are renovated. Often, as in this case, other houses in the same block either have not been renovated or are in the process of being renovated. As yet, the mother has not secured "safe" housing for herself and her children.

Although the 16-mo loss to follow-up in this case is far from optimal, it illustrates a frequent and difficult problem. It also points out that screening tests must be repeated at rather frequent intervals among children who move about in substandard rental property. It is considered that prognosis must be guarded in this case.

Lead Absorption in a Child at Home during Removal of Leaded Paint

The next case illustrates two problems which are associated with the abatement process itself and are, unfortunately, common in our experience.

Case 4. The serial PbB and FEP data in Figure 4 show the course of an infant who remained at home during the burning, scraping and sanding of old lead-containing paint. When this child was first tested, PbB was normal (25 μg); however, there was evidence of associated iron deficiency, which presumably, was responsible for the elevation in FEP observed. This 15-mo-old infant's older preschool siblings had been tested and found to have increased lead absorption; consequently, orders were issued to abate lead hazards in the home. The abatement process was being carried out during the fortnight prior to this child's admission, at which time PbB had increased from 25 μg to 65 μg and FEP had risen sharply to more than 700 μg/dl erythrocytes. After a 2-wk course of chelation therapy in hospital, the child was discharged home upon receipt of word that the lead hazards had been completely abated and all the debris removed. On this advice, outpatient treatment with oral d-penicillamine was continued; however, the child's subsequent course indicated that this was in error. There was a sharp rise in PbB during the fortnight immediately following discharge from 22 to 47 μg Pb. Reinspection of the home revealed that all hazards had not, in fact, been removed, which apparently explained the sharp rise in PbB. It should be noted in Figure 4 that this sharp rise was not reflected in FEP, which continued to decline. At this point, the family moved into modern "lead free" public housing. The subsequent course shows a continued decline in PbB and FEP although there was a brief rise during the few wk immediately following the cessation of d-penicillamine therapy.

Fig. 4. Changes in PbB and FEP in an infant during deleading of an old home. Infant remained in home during burning, scraping and sanding of old lead containing paint as PbB and FEP levels increased dramatically during a fortnight of intense exposure. Infant was hospitalized and treated with chelating agents, medicinal iron and prophylactic amounts of copper and zinc. The rise in PbB from 22-47 μg during fortnight immediately after discharge indicated incomplete abatement of hazards. When this was found, family moved quickly to modern "lead-free" public housing. PbB and FEP subsequently decreased (Chisolm and Barltrop, 1979).

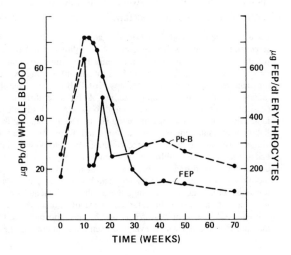

We have had extraordinary difficulty in our attempt to achieve coordination of medical treatment (chelation therapy) and abatement of lead hazards in the home to reduce the child's level of exposure, as illustrated by this case. The hazard of having young children in the home during the burning and sanding of the old paint, which creates a substantial increase in fine particulate lead, remains largely unappreciated by either public health authorities, property owners or the parents of the children. Parents seem to think, despite strong advice to the contrary, that if the child is out of the house during the actual work, it is perfectly safe for them to return to spend the night. Some parents who do appreciate this point can find no alternate housing for the child while this process is being carried out. In other instances, such as this, attention has been focused on those with increased lead absorption without regard to children found to have "normal" PbB at the time of testing. I am even aware of one situation in which a home was being deleaded on account of one child, while cousins residing in the same residence were apparently unknown to the health authorities, who ordered the abatement. This particular case came to light when one of the cousins showed up in a local hospital with early acute lead encephalopathy with convulsions (PbB = 140 μg). It is a hard and fast rule in our clinic that all children must return to the clinic within 2 wk after discharge from the hospital, because of the frequency with which spikes in PbB are detected and reinspection of the dwelling shows that all lead hazards (scaling lead containing paint) have not been removed. Prognosis in the case shown in Figure 4 probably is good in view of the short duration of excessive lead absorption and the fact that the family moved to a low lead environment.

Interplay of Housing and Extended Family Resources

This case is chosen to illustrate the impact on lead absorption of the availability of housing among extended families with limited resources.

Case 5. Patients 1 and 2 in Figure 5 are siblings. Patient 1 was 26 mos of age when first screened for lead in a well-baby clinic. After follow-up at that site, PbB was increased to over 50 μg and the child was referred to the Kennedy Institute, where he was first seen 2 mos later at 34 mos of age. PbB was 50 μg and FEP (not shown) was highly elevated. He was admitted to the inpatient service for chelation therapy. His PbB dropped sharply during chelation therapy, as indicated by the solid portion of the line. At the time of the initial referral, his younger sibling (Patient 2), age 6 mos, was also found to have a modestly elevated PbB (34 μg). During this first admission it was learned from the Health Department that there was a substantial amount of flaking lead-containing paint in the home and, furthermore, that it was unlikely that the landlord would move quickly to correct the violation. What to do with the 6-mo-old sibling? The mother had a sister in a small public housing unit who was able to take one, but not both, of the children until mother could find suitable housing for herself and both of the children. Therefore, the 6-mo-old infant moved in with the aunt and his blood lead level rather promptly decreased. It has remained within the normal range during the subsequent 18 mos of follow-up. Unfortunately, the older sibling had to be returned to the old home. Again, his PbB increased during the subsequent 2 mos from 28 to 57 μg and he was rehospitalized for a second course of chelation therapy. No progress whatsoever had been made in abating the lead hazards within the home.

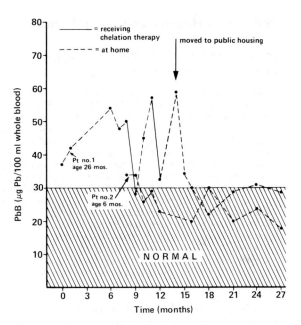

Fig. 5. Serial changes PbB in two siblings as related to housing. Patient 1, the older sibling, was treated twice in hospital as indicated by the solid segments of the line showing trends in that patient's PbB. Patient 2, the younger sibling, was first tested at the age of 6 mos when the older sibling was hospitalized and sent immediately to stay with an aunt in public "lead-free" housing. At the time that patient 1's PbB spiked for a third time, the family, including both siblings, moved to public housing. Patient 1's PbB promptly declined without additional chelation therapy. The shaded portion of the figure indicates the "normal" PbB range.

Indeed, the description of this home strongly suggested that it was not worth rehabilitating. At the time of the first admission, Social Service began an intensive effort to secure public housing for this mother and her children. When the child returned 6 wk after the second course of chelation therapy, blood lead had risen from 33 to 59 µg; however, as indicated in Figure 5 the mother had secured public housing and was to move in within 48 hr. Subsequent to this move, PbB decreased spontaneously to 30 µg Pb over the next 8 wk. During the ensuing 11 mos of follow-up it has fluctuated on a seasonal basis as shown in Figure 5. The spike in PbB to 30 µg in Patient 2 indicated at the 18th month of follow-up is associated with visits of that child to a relative in an old housing area. When the mother stopped this practice, PbB in Patient 2 remained within the normal range during the ensuing 9 mos of follow-up.

This case illustrates the often limited resources of some families. The children's aunt was willing to take both children; however, she had room in her small apartment for one child only. Consequently, triage had to be practiced and the younger infant was selected because of his very young age for quick removal to safe housing. It seems likely that the very rapid decrease in PbB in Patient 1 following transfer to public housing was due, in part, to the prior courses of chelation therapy which had reduced to a certain extent his body lead burden. In fact, the rate of decrease is more rapid than would have been expected had no therapy ever been given.

Interplay of Housing and Social Factors

The next case is chosen to illustrate a problem that faces many working mothers; namely, how to secure adequate day care facilities for their young children.

Case 6. This infant was first tested at 12 mos of age and found to have normal PbB (28 μg) and evidence of iron deficiency as indicated by the elevated FEP value. It was learned that the mother lived in public housing where there was a day care nursery in which she could leave the infant while she was away at work. Medicinal iron was prescribed, but it seems doubtful that it was ever given on a regular basis. It was also reported by the mother that the infant had indiscriminate pica, which was confirmed by observations in the clinic. Each summer this day care nursery closed in June to reopen in September. During the summer months, the working mother had no choice but to send the child to his grandmother, who lived in old housing and apparently relegated much of the infant's supervision to his young teenage cousins. As indicated in Figure 6, both PbB and FEP rose sharply during June, July and early August, whereupon he was hospitalized for chelation therapy and institution of medicinal iron on a regular basis. This therapy is indicated by the solid portion of the bars in Figure 6. Upon discharge, the day care nursery had reopened and PbB remained between 25 and 29 μg during the subsequent 30 wk of follow-up. During this period, medicinal iron therapy was continued until FEP decreased to normal. Unfortunately, the cycle illustrated in Figure 6 was repeated during each of the two subsequent summers, during which the day care nursery closed and the mother again had to send the child to stay with the grandmother in an old house in which scaling lead paint persisted.

The data in Figures 2 and 6 illustrate the problems which working mothers face. In Case 2 the mother was able to secure adequate day care for her child, while in this instance, Case 6, the mother was not successful. Adequate day care, a most important social consideration for the working mother, would assist greatly in the medical management of the children of working mothers.

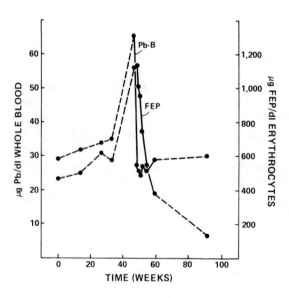

Fig. 6. Trends in PbB and FEP in relation to change in housing. During winter months, infant lived in "lead-free" public housing; however, for social reasons child had to live in old dilapidated housing during the summer. In summer PbB and FEP increased sharply as noted in the figure.

Table 3.   Serial blood lead and FEP data on retarded child with persistent pica and multiple exposures.

Age (yr)	Location	FEP	PbB	Comment
4 7/12	Home	559	54	Scaling Pb paint in home
4 8/12	1st admission	574	56	Begin chelation therapy
4 10/12	Discharge to home	386	34	Discharge to old home, abatement uncertain, no medication
5 0/12	At home	276	39	
5 5/12	2nd admission	740	74	2nd admission for chelation therapy, hazards in home abated during this admission
5 9/12	Discharge to home	270	34	
5 10/12	At home	278	40	No scaling paint in home
6 3/12	3rd admission	359	48	5-day course CaEDTA for "rebound"
		349	24	Discharge data
6 5/12	Entered special school	234	38	Special school in old mansion
6 7/12	In special school	311	55	New exposure, check school
6 8/12	4th admission	326	54	Scaling Pb paint in school
6 9/12	5th admission	516	55	Home OK, CaEDTA (5 days)
	Discharge	459	27	School closed for repairs
6 11/12	At home	414	36	Back in special school
7 1/12	At home	293	43	Back in special school
7 3/12	At home	237	38	Stabilizing

Retarded Child with Persistent Pica and Sources of Lead Outside of the Home

Many (but not all) retarded children, regardless of the primary cause of their retardation, may both be mobile and have persistent pica. The data in Table 3 illustrate such a case.

Case 7. This retarded child was first found to have lead toxicity (CDC Class III) at 55 mos of age. During the subsequent 3.5 yr of follow-up, he has been treated for lead toxicity five times as an inpatient. The fact that he has voracious pica and is rather severely retarded has been repeatedly observed in hospital. The first three courses of chelation therapy were clearly related to his residence in an old dilapidated house. Shortly after the third admission, the mother moved into a totally rehabilitated house where several inspections revealed no evidence of any lead-containing paint. Coincident with this move into apparently safe housing, the child was admitted to a special school for the retarded, which was in an old mansion. Inspection pinpointed the school, rather than the home, as a source of lead in this case. Numerous areas of interior and exterior flaking leaded paint were found in areas frequented by the children. It took about 6 mos to abate the hazards in the school. The most recent laboratory data would suggest that they may, in fact, have been abated (Table 3). Other retarded children in the special school were tested and some were found to have lead toxicity and treated.

This child illustrates a common problem, particularly among older retarded children. While many schools are of modern construction and free of lead paint hazards, a number, particularly among institutions for the retarded, are in very old buildings. A recent similar episode occurred in a 14-yr-old girl with a long history of recurrent lead poisoning, including acute lead encephalopathy about 10 years ago. In the case of the 14-yr-old girl, she was transferred from a modern school for the retarded to one which included both new and very old sections. She was in the old section. Thus, while the childhood lead poisoning prevention programs in the United States rightly place major emphasis upon the child's residence, all possible sources must be considered in the management of individual cases. In retarded children follow-up may be necessary for many years.

Urban Homesteading

Cases of plumbism and increased lead absorption are not limited to the very poor who reside in substandard rental property. Although it may be known among certain members of the medical profession that the renovation of old housing can be hazardous, this fact seems not to be generally appreciated. There is at present in the United States a rather strong trend toward urban homesteading. Those moving into and rehabilitating older homes tend to come largely from the young middle and upper economic segment of the population. The clinic receives a steady but small number of requests by these people for the testing of themselves and their young children. The following case illustrates some interesting points in this regard.

Case 8. A young mother was advised by her next-door neighbor, a biochemist working in experimental lead research, to have herself tested because she was possibly pregnant and was renovating a dwelling which was approximately 100 to 125 yr old. Mother, father and the 4-yr-old child were tested serially over a 3-mo period. The data are summarized in Table 4. The mother came, not because of concern for herself, but because she was removing old paint in her son's room. History revealed that the father was using a torch to melt the old paint, while it was

Table 4.   Young urban homesteading couple remodeling 100-yr-old home.

Family member	Weeks Post-Exposure	FEP*	PbB†
Mother	1	98	48
	2	115	41
	3	149	31
	5	129	24
	10	109	19
Father	2	65	23
	10	60	24
Child (4 yr)	1	65	30
	3	97	18
	10	87	22
Normal Values: Child		70 ± 22	<30
Adult		51 ± 14	

*FEP, μg protoporphyrin/dl erythrocytes.
†PbB, μg Pb/dl whole blood.

the mother's job to sand this down to the bare surface. History revealed that the mother had done this during the course of approximately two wk before her first blood lead test. The son and father were apparently unaffected; however, the mother showed an elevated PbB, which subsequently fell to well within the normal range as she stopped any further renovation work. The delayed response of FEP is clearly evident in the mother's case as it rose to a peak approximately two wk later and thereafter declined toward normal. After discussion with several experts in the field, the mother elected to maintain the pregnancy, which is now still in progress.

This case illustrates rather nicely the delayed response in FEP following rather short exposure. It also illustrates the dilemma that the pregnant woman faces. In this particular case the various experts that she consulted apparently considered that the risk of brief over-exposure at such an early stage in pregnancy did not pose a substantial risk; however, it was the mother who made her own decision, when all of the uncertainties were explained to her. The case illustrates another point that we have frequently observed; it is generally the sander and not the burner who shows increased lead absorption among husband and wife urban homesteading pairs. We have, in fact, encountered a few incidents of symptomatic plumbism in such cases.

Fouling One's Own Nest

An important part of the workup in the Kennedy Institute Lead Clinic is a detailed occupational history of all adult residents of the home in which the child lives. Furthermore, there is a working relationship between the clinic and occupational physicians in the community who, in turn, alertly refer the children of workers found to have elevated PbB to the clinic. The clinic, in turn, refers parents who are exposed to lead to the occupational physician.

Case 9. The data in Table 5 illustrate two such families. In Family A the worker was the index case. During the several weeks prior to testing he had developed progressively severe headache, behavioral change, anorexia, abdominal colic and intermittent vomiting. He had seen three general practitioners because of these complaints and no etiological diagnosis had been made. His wife reported that his headaches had been so severe that she had taken him to the emergency room twice in the middle of the night. This family, however, lived next door to one of the city Health Department aides working in the childhood lead poisoning program. It was she who suspected the diagnosis and referred him, his wife and children to the Kennedy Institute clinic for testing. The man worked in an automobile assembly plant, where his job was to grind down to a smooth surface the lead solder used in sealing joints between various automobile body parts. Apparently, he did shower and change his clothing before going home, but only erratically. He was referred to an occupational physician for treatment of his clinical plumbism. Fortunately, his wife and children were unaffected.

Family B presented a diagnostic puzzle to the referring physician. The 2-yr-old child was the index case in this family He lived in a nearby county where public concern had been raised over the possibility that water supplies in the county contained excessive amounts of lead. When this concern proved to be unfounded, the child was referred to the Kennedy Institute on the assumption that his increased lead absorption was due to exposure to lead-containing paints. The history, however, strongly suggested that this was not the case. The home was a newly constructed bungalow made primarily of cinderblock and synthetic building materials. The father, who had built it, said he had used only latex paints. Testing of the water, soil and paint in

Table 5.   Occupational lead poisoning family studies.

Subject	Exposure	FEP*	Blood Lead†
	Family A		
Worker	Grinding solder	757	88
Wife	—	72	23
Child, 9 1/2 yr	—	56	28
Child, 6 1/2 yr	—	65	26
	Family B		
Worker	Brass cutter	641	68
Wife	—	82	10
Child, 2 yr	—	968	52
Normal Values: Child		70 ± 22	<30
Adult		51 ± 14	

*FEP, μg protoporphyrin/dl erythrocytes.
†PbB, μg Pb/dl whole blood.

the home did not reveal any hazardous lead source. At the time of the first clinic visit, the father stated that he worked at an aluminum processing company. Specific questioning, however, indicated that he was a brass cutter. Brass may contain 5 to 10% lead. His wife volunteered the information that he came home covered from head to toe with metal filings. He usually played with the child immediately upon his arrival home before showering and changing his clothing. The wife further volunteered the information that the family car was also full of metal filings and that they frequently took the child with them in the automobile. The child was treated with chelation therapy. The parents thoroughly washed down the home and automobile with high phosphate detergents. The child spontaneously improved and has had normal lead absorption status during the ensuing two years of follow-up. This case was also reported to the Maryland Occupational Health Agency. Investigation subsequently revealed a few other men in the plant with increased lead absorption. Improvement in industrial hygiene practices in the plant followed.

These cases illustrate the importance of cooperation between pediatrician and occupational physician. Either the child or a worker may be the index case. One must also determine not only the worker's occupation but also his place of employment. Recently, in the investigation of another child with increased lead absorption, no hazardous lead sources were found within the home. The mother stated that the father was an electrician. This occupation is not ordinarily associated with hazardous lead exposure. However, this man was employed as an electrician to repair wiring in an old ship in drydock. He was working in poorly ventilated enclosed areas deep in the ship in which other workers were removing old marine lead-containing paints in the process of repairing the ship. Marine lead-containing paints may contain 70 to 80% of lead by weight. This man came home dusty in his work clothing. On our advice, he began promptly to change his work clothing and shower elsewhere. Shortly thereafter he transferred to another place where he was not exposed to lead. The child's blood lead concentration decreased spontaneously. The National Institute of Occupational

Safety and Health lists at least 110 occupations with potential exposure to lead. It behooves the physician to learn which of these lead trades may be found in his locality (Chisolm, 1978).

Summary

These cases have been chosen to illustrate the wide variety of problems that the physician managing children with increased lead absorption may encounter. Serial PbB and FEP data are necessary, not only to judge the course of lead absorption, but also to evaluate management plans and modify them according to the course of the child. In interpreting FEP-PbB pairs the question of iron deficiency must always be considered. Perhaps most important is a detailed environmental and occupational history. These provide clues which can be conveyed to the local health authority. Such clues often facilitate the identification of the major environmental lead source(s) in the child's environment. A Baltimore City Health Department nurse assigned to the lead program regularly attends the Kennedy Institute Lead Clinic sessions. Her presence greatly facilitates liaison between the agencies and should provide coordinated medical and environmental management, although as can be seen by a number of the cases cited, effective environmental management is frequently quite slow. Environmental and medical management also require close coordination with Social Service as one is often dealing with multiproblem families. The crux of the issue is the serious problem presented by substandard housing. In our view, success in management is achievable only when safe housing can be secured by the families of affected children. Although the cases just presented may seem to indicate that results are not optimal, I may say, as one who has been dealing with children with lead poisoning for almost 30 years, that there have been very substantial improvements over the years. Thirty years ago almost all of the children identified with lead poisoning were ones with acute lead encephalopathy. Today, with early screening, all but a few are clinically asymptomatic. It is strongly suspected that screening and close follow-up of those found to be at high risk has played a role in reducing substantially the numbers of children with severe forms of plumbism.

References

Albert, R.E., Shore, R. E., Sayers, A.J., Strehlow, C., Kneip, T.J., Pasternack, B.S., Friedhoff, A.J., Covan, F. and Cimino, J.A., 1974. Follow-up of children overexposed to lead. Environ Health Perspec 7:33–40.

Bradley, J.E., Powell, A.E., Niermann, W.,

McGrady, K.R. and Kaplan E., 1956. The incidence of abnormal blood levels of lead in a metropolitan pediatric clinic with observation on the value of coproporphyrinuria as screening test. J Pediat 49:1–6.

Center for Disease Control. 1978. Preventing lead poisoning in young children: A statement by the Center for Disease Control. J Pediat 93:709–720.

Chisolm, J.J. Jr. 1975. Screening for Pediatric Lead Poisoning. Arch Ind Hyg Toxi 26 (Suppl. 1):61–79.

Chisolm, J.J. Jr. 1978. Fouling one's own nest. Pediatrics 62:614–617.

Chisolm, J.J., Jr. and Barltrop, D. 1979. Recognition and management of children with increased lead absorption. Arch Dis Childh 54:249–262.

Chisolm, J.J., Jr., Barrett, M.B. and Mellits, E.D. 1979. Evidence for interactions among lead, zinc and iron in children. Arch Ind Hyg Toxi 30 (suppl. 1):117–122.

Chisolm, J.J., Jr. and Brown, D.H. 1975. Micro-scale photofluorometric determination of "free erythrocyte porphyrin" (protoporphyrin IX). Clin Chem 21:1669–1682.

Chisolm, J.J., Jr. and Brown, D.H. 1979. Micromethod for zinc protoporphyrin in erythrocytes: Including new data on the absorptivity of zinc protoporphyrin and new observations in neonates and sickle cell disease. Biochem Med 22:214–237.

Chisolm, J.J., Jr., Mellits, E.D. and Barrett, M.B. 1976. Interrelationships among blood lead concentration, quantitative daily ALA-U and urinary lead output following calcium EDTA. In Effects and Dose-Response Relationships of Toxic Metals. Nordberg, G.F., Ed. Elsevier Scientific Publishing, New York. pp. 416–433.

Jugo, S., Maljkovic, T. and Kostial, K., 1975. Influence of chelating agents on the gastrointestinal absorption of lead. Toxi Applied Pharmacol 34:259–263.

Kaplan. E. and McDonald, J. 1942. Amer J Pub Hlth 32:481–486.

Piomelli, S., Young, P. and Gay, G. 1973. A micromethod for free erythrocyte porphyrins: The FEP test. J Lab Clin Med 81:932–940.

Pueschel, S.M., Kopito, L. and Schwachman, H., 1972. Children with an increased lead burden. A screening and follow-up study. JAMA 222:462–466.

Reiders, F. 1954. Effect of oral Na₂Ca ethylenediamine tetraacetate on urinary and fecal excretion of lead in rabbits. Fed Proc 13:397.

Rummo, J.H., (1974), Intellectual and behavioral effects of lead poisoning in children. Ph.D. thesis, University of North Carolina, Chapel Hill, N.C., Ann Arbor, Mich., University of Mich. Microfilms, as cited in 1977 EPA-600/8-77-017, Chapter 11, p 11–21.

World Health Organization (WHO). 1977. Environmental Health Criteria 3, Lead. Geneva.

19. Implications of Newer Data for Screening and Evaluation of Children

Vernon N. Houk

Civilization, in seeking to improve the quality of life, has become increasingly dependent upon rapidly evolving knowledge and technology. In the last century scientific knowledge of the physical environment and its impact on man has grown dramatically. With each new discovery we become more aware of hazards. In our eagerness to improve the quality of life, we have been highly successful in creating an environment conducive to human illness. Hazardous substances in our home, work and recreational environments are the rule rather than the exception.

Lead toxicity is a classic among environmentally induced diseases. Because of its low melting point (327°C), conductibility, malleability, availability and weathering resistance, lead has always been regarded as a highly desirable metal. However, it has been discovered that some medical conditions are caused by the inhalation or ingestion of leaded substances. Symptoms such as a metallic taste in the mouth, colic, constipation and weakness of extensor muscle groups are described in adult populations involved in lead-related industries. Descriptions such as that of the Endemial Colic of Devonshire (Baker, 1767) highlighted the impact of lead contamination in our food chain.

While our knowledge about the adverse effects of lead was increasing, the annual use of lead also continued to increase dramatically. Lead was used in glazing pottery, storage batteries and fuel. When mixed with an appropriate oil base, it was found to be highly desirable as a paint. Eventually, the increasing use of lead enhanced the contamination of the environment so that individuals other than workers in lead-related industries were exposed to increasing amounts of lead.

As industrial technologies found new uses for lead, medical knowledge also advanced. The literature is replete with descriptions of the symptoms of lead poisoning. Among the milder symptoms and signs are fatigue, pallor, malaise, appetite loss, irritability, sleep disturbance, sudden behavioral change and developmental regression. More severe lead symptoms are clumsiness, ataxia, weakness, abdominal pain, persistent vomiting, constipation and changes in consciousness which can presage encephalopathy. The tissues and organs most severely affected by lead are the bone marrow, kidney and brain. It is also now known that most children with lead toxicity are without the aforementioned symptoms.

Factors which affect the absorption of lead have been described. We know that younger children absorb a greater portion of the lead available to them than do older ones. The composition of diet is important. Increased dietary unsaturated fat and decreased dietary intake of calcium, iron and possibly other nutrients enhance the absorption of lead from the intestine in experimental animals.

Investigators have evaluated the impact of lead upon man through laboratory analyses of feces, hair, urine, blood, cerebral spinal fluid and teeth. We have developed techniques to measure excretion of delta-aminolevulinic acid in urine (ALA-U), excretion of coproporphyrin in urine (CPU) and inhibition of delta-aminolevulinate dehydratase (ALA-D) activity, as assayed in vitro in circulating erythrocytes and erythrocyte protoporphyrin.

Technologic advances in the use of lead have increased the availability of this contaminant and the total body lead burden of man. This increase results from the complex sum of many different vectors including air, dust, dirt and diet. The relative contribution of each source is not wholly understood. Logic dictates that every effort be made to reduce the individual's total exposure to lead. This is particularly critical for children, inasmuch as permanent neurologic damage is incurred if neurotoxic insult occurs during brain growth and development. The growth spurt begins during the sixth month of pregnancy and continues until the fourth year postpartum. As the child becomes ambulatory and explores his environment, the potential for increased lead absorption is enhanced. Of all the lead vectors in our environment, lead-based paint constitutes the major high-dose source and is the most common cause of overt lead poisoning in children.

Prior to the evolution of screening programs, childhood lead poisoning was diagnosed and treated on an individual acute care basis. A comatose child was brought to a hospital where the attending physician diagnosed the child on the basis of observed symptoms, x-ray findings revealing lead lines in the long bones or chips in the gut, basophilic stippling and a history elicited from the parent. The child was hospitalized, chelated, reported in some instances and most often released to return to the living environment from which he came. This process is analogous to controlling poliomyelitis with the iron lung.

There had to be a better way than treating children after they had developed overt signs and symptoms of severe lead poisoning. Preventive medicine and public health practice dictate early intervention in a disease process if adverse consequences are to be avoided. Consequently, tests for elemental lead were employed for both diagnostic and screening purposes in several major cities of this country. The results indicated that a significant number of children with evidence of high lead absorption were asymptomatic. Environmental epidemiologic investigations continued to incriminate lead-based paint as one of the major vectors. Lead poisoning was considered to be a problem primarily of the inner part of large cities in the so-called "Lead Belt" of the Northeast.

The Surgeon General's statement, "Medical Aspects of Childhood Lead Poisoning (1970)," focused attention on the problem of lead poisoning. With the passage of the Lead-Based Paint Poisoning Prevention Act (PL 91-695), a grant program was established by the Federal Government to assist communities in screening children at high risk of lead poisoning. From 1972 to 1979, communities receiving Federal support for screening activities reported testing approximately 2.5 million children and identifying 170,735 children with lead toxicity. It is now known that when children under the age of 6 yr who live in a hazardous environment containing excess lead are tested, 3 to 20% will be identified as having metabolic effects due to elevated blood lead levels. This is true whether the children live in the East, West, North or South or in a rural or urban setting. It is our estimate that 1% of all children ages 1 to 5 yr have lead toxicity. Yet, each year we test only about 500,000 of the 15 million children in this age group.

Just as technology created the problem, technology has also brought us a means to identify children with lead toxicity and to institute activities to reduce the child's risk of lead poisoning. Our problem now resides in the application of technology and the mobilization of resources through a united effort to ameliorate this situation. We cannot expect to undo centuries of environmental abuse in the immediate future. We can, however, take direct and positive steps to reduce the total exposure of children and to assure that all children receive appropriate screening and the required medical and environmental services when lead toxicity is identified. It is only through a total effort that we can hope to prevent the devastating neurologic effects of lead exposure.

The Consumer Product Safety Commission (CPSC) has lowered the permissible lead content of paint to 0.06% by weight for paint intended for child-related purposes. Similar regulatory activities have been instituted by the Food and Drug Administration (FDA), resulting in lower lead levels in processed food. The Environmental Protection Agency (EPA) has established criteria for allowable air lead levels. The Occupational Safety and Health Administration (OSHA) has also issued new recommended standards for occupational exposure to inorganic lead.

Many of these activities will have a long-term effect in reducing background lead exposure of children in our society. They will, however, do little to eliminate existing lead contamination in our environment. The economics involved in total environmental lead decontamination mount into the hundreds of billions of dollars. Thus, although the Department of Housing and Urban Development (HUD), the Veterans Administration (VA), the Farmers Home Administration (FHA) and the Department of Defense (DOD) have addressed the problem of lead paint hazards, millions of dwellings remain contaminated.

We must not approach the childhood lead poisoning problem categorically by playing one lead vector against another, nor should we state that the situation is so large and the consequences so great that a group of experts should be convened to investigate, evaluate, contemplate and report on the need for future research. Rather, let each of us do what we do best, coordinating our efforts. We must remember that the quality of life begins in childhood and that we must start where we can produce long-term results.

It has long been known that lead exposure results in anemia. One of the first effects of increased lead exposure is on the hematopoietic system. The resulting multiple interferences in the formation of hemoglobin are manifested in excess protoporphyrin. With the advent of a simple optical method for erythrocyte protoporphyrin (EP) determinations we can now analyze a drop of blood quickly and inexpensively, without the concern for contamination experienced in blood lead analysis. Abnormal EP levels are also observed in iron deficiency with or without frank anemia, allowing identification of the exhaustion of iron reserves before anemia is manifest.

The development of a simple means to measure erythrocyte protoporphyrin now makes it economically feasible to screen all children ages 1 to 5 for lead toxicity and iron deficiency. I would propose that our national course of action to address pediatric lead toxicity be as follows.

The Federal Government must continue to limit the addition of lead to our environment. Significant steps have been made in this regard through issuance of regulations and guidelines by EPA, CPSC, HUD, FDA and OSHA.

Lead poisoning prevention activities require laboratories with demonstrated proficiency in analyzing blood lead and erythrocyte protoporphyrin samples. This capacity must be made available throughout the country. Instrumentation for onsite EP determinations can be acquired for less than $3500 and allows initial screening to be completed before the child leaves the screening site. The Centers for Disease Control (CDC) will continue to offer proficiency testing services on a monthly basis to laboratories serving lead poisoning prevention programs. The quarterly proficiency testing program will be offered to all laboratories participating in interstate commerce. However, many states should proceed to develop their own intensive proficiency testing services.

Federal programs supporting services to children must remove programmatic barriers and actively encourage routine EP screening for all children ages 1 to 5. Significant progress has been made as evidenced in recent guidance documents released by the Health Services Administration and Health Care Financing Administration. The Department of Agriculture's Women, Infants and Children (WIC) Program now recognizes the erythrocyte protoporphyrin test as an allowable screening procedure for iron deficiency. Many Federal agencies are meeting to address the problem of lead toxicity and to coordinate policy and services.

The various academies of the medical profession must encourage their members to pursue aggressively screening of children for lead toxicity. This will involve upgrading the academies' and the practicing physicians' awareness of the magnitude, nature and consequences of lead toxicity and familiarizing them with current technology and recommendations in this field. Most physicians were trained to recognize the symptoms of lead poisoning. Few, however, are trained in current methods of recognizing the asymptomatic child. Unless the entire medical community realizes that all children are at some risk of lead toxicity and seeks to identify asymptomatic children with lead toxicity, some children requiring care will go undetected.

We should encourage the development or modification of public health reporting requirements so that all children identified with lead toxicity are reported to the state or local health department. There are two major reasons for this action. First, a child who is asymptomatic requires environmental epidemiologic services and hazard reduction as much as a child who presents with severe symptoms. Second, unless instances of asymptomatic lead toxicity are brought to the attention of state and local government, lead toxicity will continue to remain a "silent epidemic."

On the state and local level the health care delivery system, both public and private, must be prepared to deliver quality diagnostic and follow-up services to children identified with lead toxicity. This implies establishment of a system with monitoring capabilities and an increase in communication among the screening, medical and environmental segments of the delivery system.

On the state and local level, environmental epidemiologic services must be provided to identify lead hazards in the environment of children with lead toxicity. The methodology and technology to do this are available. However, the majority of communities in this country have not developed the expertise or instrumentation necessary to provide the service. The CDC has established a demonstration program in cooperation with the Detroit, Michigan, Health Department to train managers and environmentalists in hazard identification and reduction methodologies.

States and communities should develop laws and regulations governing the removal of lead-based paint hazards. Such laws must be realistic in their requirements, but must be designed so that children with lead toxicity can be protected from further high-dose lead exposure. Without the assurance that environmental intervention will occur, medical management is incomplete.

Lead hazard abatement is a labor-intensive activity. Newer and more cost-efficient means of hazard reduction must be developed. In this regard, the Department of Housing and Urban Development is currently evaluating methodologies which offer potential in reducing the economic impact on the property owner required to reduce lead-based paint hazards. The CDC also has worked with the Internal Revenue Service. As a result, the owner occupant of a house can now deduct the cost of removing lead-based paint as a medical expense when the removal is ordered by a physician. Other assistance in hazard reduction is available to communities from a variety of sources such as Community Development Funds, Housing Rehabilitation Funds and Comprehensive Employment and Training Act (CETA). We must all work to develop local commitment to hazard reduction.

A coordinated focus on the State and local level must be developed. Effective identification of children with lead toxicity and provision of appropriate medical and environmental services require bringing together diverse programs and expertise. The Lead-Based Paint Poisoning Prevention Act has enabled many communities to develop a coordinated program. To assist other community and state child health providers in developing appropriate systems and a coordinated program, the CDC maintains a demonstration program in Louisville, Kentucky, where managers and physicians can receive practical orientation in the various components of a childhood lead poisoning prevention program. Technical and managerial consultation is also available from the CDC.

The prevention of neurologic sequelae associated with increased absorption of lead can be accomplished through the total removal of lead from our environment. However, until the societal commitment exists to remove high-dose vectors of lead in paint and lead in soil as a result of contamination from lead paint, automotive emissions, industrial pollution and previous land use, we must rely on early detection and intervention in the disease process. An effective approach to the problem must involve the combined efforts of Federal, state, and local governments working in concert with the private medical community and industry. Resources are available if we elect to give pediatric lead toxicity priority. There must be a commitment to apply the technology we now have through a coordinated effort to remove this man-made threat to the quality of life for the Nation's children.

References

Baker, G. 1767. An essay concerning the cause of the endemial colic of Devonshire. Reprinted by the Delta Omega Society, 1958. Reproduced courtesy of The Royal College of Physicians, London.

Barltrop, D. and Khoo, H.E. 1975. The influence of nutritional factors on lead absorption. Postgrad Med J 51:795.

Benson, P.F. and Chisolm, J.J., Jr. 1960. A reliable qualitative use coproporphyrin test for lead intoxication in young children. J Pediatr 56:759.

Chisolm, J.J., Jr. and Brown, D.H. 1975. Micro-scale photofluorometric determination of "free erythrocyte porphyrin" (Protoporphyrin IX). Clin Chem 21:1669.

Chisolm, J.J., Jr., Mellits, E.D. and Barrett, M.D. 1976. Interrelationships among blood lead concentration, quantitative daily ALA-U and urinary lead output following calcium

EDTA. In Effects and Dose-Response Relationships of Toxic Metals, G.F. Norberg, Ed. Elsevier, Amsterdam.

Committee on Toxicology. 1976. Recommendations for the prevention of lead poisoning in Children. National Academy of Science. National Research Council, Washington.

Granick, J.L., Sassa, S., Granick, S., Levere, R.D. and Kappas, A. 1973. Studies in lead poisoning. II. Correlation between the ratio of activated to inactivated δ-aminolevulinic acid dehydratase of whole blood and the blood lead level. Biochem Med 8:149.

Health Care Financing Administration. Action Transmittal: HCFA-AT-78-59(MMB). July 7, 1978.

Internal Revenue Bulletin No. 1979-9. Medical expenses; lead poisoning; removal of lead-based paint. Rev Rul 79:66:8.

Joint Statement: Lead Poisoning in Children. 1979. Bureau of Community Health Services and Center for Disease Control.

Kammholz, L.P., Thatcher, G., Blodgett, F. M. and Good, T.A. 1972. Rapid protoporphyrin quantitation for detection of lead poisoning. Pediatrics 50:625.

Needleman, H.L. 1977. Exposure to lead: sources and effects. N Engl J Med 297:17.

Pinto, L., Esposito, L. and Nobili, B. 1977. Diagnostic methods in iron deficiency states. Comparative data on free protoporphyrins of erythrocytes in iron deficiency states and in thalassemia. Pediatria 85(2):291–310.

Piomelli, S., Davidow, B., Guinee, V.F., Young, P. and Gay, G. 1973. The FEP (free erythrocyte porphyrins) test: A screening micromethod for lead poisoning. Pediatrics 51:254.

Rabinowitz, M.B., Wetherill, G.W. and Kopple, J.D. 1976. Kinetic analysis of lead metabolism in healthy humans. J Clin Invest 58:260.

Sassa, S., Granick, J.L., Granick, S., Kappas, A. and Levere, R.D. 1973. Studies in lead poisoning. I. Microanalysis of erythrocyte protoporphyrin levels of spectrofluorometry in the detection of chronic lead intoxication in the subclinical range. Biochem Med 8:135.

Sayre, J.W., Charney, E., Vostal, J. and Pless, I.B. 1974. House and hand dust as a potential source of childhood lead exposure. Am J Dis Child 127:167.

Six, K.M. and Goyer, R.A. 1972. The influence of iron deficiency on tissue content and toxicity of ingested lead in the rat. J Lab Clin Med 79:128.

Spencer, S.M. 1972. America's tragic "silent epidemic." Reader's Digest, April, 1972.

Stockman, J.A., III, Weiner, L.S., Simon, G.E., Stuart, M.J. and Oski, F.A. 1975. The measurement of free erythrocyte protoporphyrin (FEP) as a simple means of distinguishing iron deficiency from beta-thalassemia trait in subjects with microcytosis. J Lab Clin Med 85(1):113–119.

Vostal, J.J., Taves, E., Sayre, J.W. and Charney, E. 1974. Lead analysis of house dust: A method for the detection of another source of lead exposure in inner city children. Environ Health Persp 7:91.

20. Research Needs

Robert A. Goyer

My involvement in lead toxicity has been largely experimental so I am going to confine my comments to approaches to experimental studies that I think are needed. The views presented here are my own and do not reflect policy of the National Institute of Environmental Health Sciences. I will comment about four topics.

Central Nervous System

It has been implied repeatedly in the presentations that we need a specific indicator of lead toxicity of the central nervous system. Even in a child who has a presumed effect, the effects are nonspecific and there are always questions about how much is due to lead and how much is due to other things. Why don't we have an ideal marker? I think there are several problems. One is that there has not been a good experimental model. I do not suggest that there is going to be one that is ideal. The brain does not have an excretory function like that of the kidney or the liver, so it is difficult to determine what is going on in the brain at any particular time. I think that, in spite of all the difficulties, modern neurobiology has tools to bring to the problem of central nervous system effects of lead that have not yet been applied. Furthermore, I think that rather than grope for nonspecific effects, hoping to find something that is going to work, it may be time to go back and do some very basic things.

I am not aware that lead has actually been localized in various parts of the brain in the refined way that our current abilities of analyzing lead would permit. If this were done, one could look at those parts of the brain and ask what the function is that might be affected. There is enough evidence to say that there are focal concentrations of lead in the brain, particularly in the toxic brain (Stowe et al., 1973). We might ask what functional effect is expected or what biochemical effect might be expected. I am not suggesting what would be found; I am simply proposing this as an approach.

Heme Metabolism

We know a great deal about the effects of lead on heme metabolism. It is now known that in lead toxicity heme binds with zinc rather than with iron and that zinc hemoglobin results (Lamola and Yamane, 1974). I do not think that there have been many studies beyond that, but it is doubtful that hemoglobin containing zinc heme binds oxygen in the way that iron hemoglobin does. I think it would be very simple for people with the right tools to measure the oxygen-carrying capacity of zinc containing heme. This might be particularly interesting in patients with sickle disease. I know that one of Dr. Chisolm's patients has homozygous sickle disease and has had pronounced effects from lead exposure. It is from the observations made in the few cases with pronounced effects that we get hints about what to look for when a pathologic effect is present to a lesser degree. The effect I would expect from zinc hemoglobin would be a relative hypoxia. This might contribute also to the central nervous system effect.

Reproduction

The need for more knowledge about reproductive fitness comes out of the growing concern that lead affects not only the fetus but also the gametes of the lead-exposed person. I think that now that we have a large group of children treated for lead poisoning in the past, and we know a lot about the level of their lead burden during childhood, it is advisable to follow these people into adulthood for reproductive fitness. This would be particularly appropriate in the female because ova are formed in utero and are fairly mature within the first year of life. I am aware of some as yet unpublished work indicating that ova in experimental animals are reduced in number and size, although nothing is known about functional changes. I do not think we need to wait until all the studies in the rat are complete. We probably have enough information to design an epidemiologic study of children with a past history of lead toxicity to describe their reproductive fitness.

Chelation Therapy

My last topic concerns some experimental studies on chelation therapy of lead toxicity in the rat. These studies were performed a few years ago while I was at the University of Western Ontario. My colleague, Dr. Cherian, was very interested in metal binding of various substances. He did some in vitro work with naturally occurring carboxylic acids. Carboxyl groups have a great affinity for lead and he found that ascorbic acid had a very strong affinity for lead. On the other hand, lactic, citric and succinic acids had virtually no chelating ability. Ascorbic acid had none when it was injected intraperitoneally, but it was quite effective when given orally. We designed an experiment, repeated it twice and published the results of the replication (Goyer and Cherian, 1979). There is a synergistic effect between ascorbic acid and edathamil calcium disodium (EDTA). I think it is important to know more about the effectiveness of ascorbic acid as a chelating agent for metals because it is a naturally occurring substance and can be bought off the drug store shelf in large quantities. Secondly, the combined therapy of EDTA and ascorbic acid might be interesting to measure in some children, although it would be hard to control the cases in the same way in which experimental studies are conducted. Finally, chelation therapy is not a satisfactory substitute for preventive medicine but, when it is needed, we should have the most effective therapy available.

References

Goyer, R.A. and Cherian, M.G. 1979. Ascorbic acid and EDTA treatment of lead toxicity in rats. Life Sciences 24:433–438

Lamola, A.A. and Yamane, T. 1974. Zinc protoporphyrin in the erythrocytes of patients with lead toxicity and iron deficiency anemia. Science 186:936–938.

Stowe, H.D., Goyer, R.A., Krigman, M.R., Wilson, M. and Cates, M. 1973. Experimental oral lead toxicity in young dogs. Arch Path 95:106–116.

21. Some Practical Problems and Solutions in Lead Poisoning Prevention Programs: An Overview of the Conference

Walter J. Rogan

Introduction

An enormous amount of information in some very good papers has been presented at this meeting. I will try to highlight those points that have the most practical impact on actual practice.

Case Finding versus Case Treatment

Dr. Lin-Fu pointed out that effective case finding is not enough; only a small percentage of children identified as at high risk of lead poisoning actually end up being treated appropriately (Chapter 1). There are at least two reasons for this. The first is an understandable reluctance on the part of the child's provider to treat an asymptomatic patient or to refer him to the university medical center for treatment. This is a problem particularly when rural cases are found and when treatment facilities are distant. The second reason is that there is often poor coordination between those responsible for case finding and those responsible for

201

treatment. One typical sequence might be an asymptomatic child found on screening to have a blood lead of 40 μg/100 cc. That child may be referred to a practitioner with little more information than the blood lead value, and the practitioner may differ from the health department in the aggressiveness with which he deals with that child. Responsibility for follow-up after referral tends to get blurred, and ultimate disposition may depend more on the curiosity of the parents about the abnormal test than on the adequacy of the treatment. This type of situation is avoided if good, effective communication takes place between referring agencies and practitioners. The goals of both are really the same, prevention of lead poisoning, but agreement on tactics and responsibilities is necessary. Once lines of communication are open, they need to be kept open, so that if questions arise, such as those regarding the latest guidelines and the identification of a good secondary referral center or resource person, they can be answered. The important point is that the referral process is one of the most vulnerable in terms of loss to follow-up and that good communication can ameliorate this problem.

Toxicity and Dose Response

Dr. Hammond (Chapter 2) showed the curvilinear relationship between external dose of lead and blood lead level, and pointed out that the curve gets less steep as it ascends. This offers some reassurance in cases of high exposure. However, the steep early part of the curve implies good absorption at low doses and consequently ubiquitous, if low, blood lead levels.

Dr. Goyer (Chapter 3) mentioned the wide variety of tests that are abnormal in lead intoxication. This is a reflection of the various toxicities of the metal and of the toxicologist's interest in measuring them. However, the availability of these tests does not mean they have a place in routine screening, treatment and follow-up. In fact, their inconstant relation to one another probably means they should be avoided. Effective screening and treatment can be done with free erythrocyte protoporphyrin (FEP), zinc protoporphyrin (ZPP), blood lead and urine lead; other tests should be left to the researcher. Dr. Goyer's other point was the susceptibility of the male gamete to lead. Remember that reproduction is a cycle, starting arbitrarily with the ability of adults to conceive at will, through gestation of normal term offspring, successful lactation, lack of childhood morbidity and mortality and ultimately successful reproduction by the offspring. Lead interferes with virtually all of these steps. It produces oligospermia and teratospermia (Lancranjan et al., 1975) and spontaneous abortion (Nogaki, 1958) in adults, crosses the placenta and intoxicates the fetus (Angle and McIntire, 1964) and, of course, produces childhood morbidity and mortality. The late effects of lead

intoxication on subsequent fertility have not yet been studied. However, some of the children followed in lead poisoning programs are now in their reproductive years and research on their reproductive capacity has yet to be done. I think it biologically plausible that some effects may be seen, but as yet we have no data.

"Critical Effects" and Clinical Disease

Dr. Chisolm (Chapter 18) spoke of critical effects and this concept needs clarification. First, a critical effect is not necessarily a clinical endpoint. It is an effect sought by the toxicologist in his search for points on the dose/response curve. The most obvious of such points is the LD-50, the dose at which half the experimental animals die. For lead, a number of responses have been shown, e.g., death, anemia, protoporphyrinemia, coproporphyrinuria and inhibition of the enzyme amino levulenate dehydratase (ALA-D). The "critical" effect is the one whose dose/response curve begins closest to the origin, i.e., occurs at the lowest dose. For lead, the current critical effect is inhibition of heme synthesis in erythroid cells in the bone marrow, as reflected by elevation of erythrocyte protoporphyrin. Regulators use critical effects as a basis for measures such as allowable levels and thus a great deal of attention is paid to whether a given phenomenon is or is not a critical effect. A critical effect need not be a symptom, sign or clinically definable illness. It simply needs to be a dose-related outcome showing that biologically significant exposure has taken place. The confusion arises when physicians are asked to treat patients whose sole manifestation of exposure is the critical effect, i.e., an elevation of FEP or ZPP accompanied by a high blood lead. In such cases, we are not just treating a laboratory abnormality, we are preventing the occurrence of encephalopathy and its sequellae in a child at high risk and are alerted to the fact that the child's environment contains too much lead and needs to be modified. This point needs emphasis, for it will help maintain good communication between case finders and providers.

Critical effects are thus signals of untoward exposure, but why is a central nervous system (CNS) critical effect emphasized? There is strong clinical suspicion that lead is active on the CNS at doses that do not produce encephalopathy. In order to evaluate such toxicity, however, we are currently forced to use time consuming, expensive methods such as intelligence testing or teacher/parent evaluations of behavior. Studies using such endpoints are always controversial and demand extraordinary investigator commitment, funds, time and method development. A biochemical marker of CNS injury would ease enormously the problems of interpretation and feasibility of study. In addition, if such a marker were a critical effect, i.e., if it responded in a dose-related fashion at a lower level than heme synthesis, then it could become the new focus of regulation.

Thus Dr. Chisolm's work (see p. 211) with homovanillic acid and vanillyl mandelic acid excretion in mild lead intoxication is both exciting and promising.

Dr. Chisolm made another point that deserves emphasis. Of all current tests available, FEP or ZPP is most useful for case finding or screening and blood lead most useful for confirmation and follow-up. This simple scheme is the most interpretable and is practical and productive even in middle class private practice (Dine, 1979).

Pregnancy Outcome and the IQ/Behavior Issue

Although not addressed specifically in a formal paper, the issue of lead and pregnancy came up often enough to deserve attention. The following recommendations seem reasonable, although they may not represent the consensus of the faculty. First, prenatal care should include an occupational history from both parents and also from any adults who come into the house. "Fouling the nest," Dr. Chisolm's term for occupational chemicals brought home on work clothes or other fomites (Chisolm, 1978), is a well described source of chemical intoxication of children. Second, habitual spontaneous abortion, or even a first spontaneous abortion, should call for an occupational history, and perhaps a ZPP, FEP or blood lead if exposure cannot be ruled out. Again, both parents should be questioned. The third issue is really more a question than a recommendation. When is the appropriate time to educate parents about environmental and occupational hazards to their children? At some point, parents should be told about the necessity of occupational hygiene, about paint hazards and about other environmental problems in the same way that they are informed about prevention of poisoning. Children are more susceptible to chemical intoxication than adults, so the absence of illness in the parent is not proof that excess exposure to the child is not taking place through work clothes, tools, paint or straightforward exposure while in utero or lactating. I suggest prenatal visits as the appropriate time to talk about this.

There was also considerable discussion about the significance of the relatively small changes in intelligence quotient (IQ) related to lead burden, reported by Needlemen et al. (1979). Specifically, the discussion centered on whether more frankly retarded children would be found because of this kind of exposure. There are three salient points here. First, the severe mental retardation following lead encephalopathy is very likely due to a mixture of the toxic effect of lead and the nonspecific aftermath of any CNS disaster, and no one proposes that we simply extrapolate arithmetically down the level/response curve to arrive at the effects of low levels. Point two, however, is that any agent that shifts a population IQ mean downward by an arbitrary amount will perforce increase the number in the population found below any specific cutoff point, if the simplistic assumption is made that the distribution remains similarly shaped. Thus, if the distribution shifts three points, a greater number of children will now be below 70, or 60, or whatever criterion. The third point is that this is a population-based epidemiologic phenomenon, not a patient-based clinical one. Dr. Graef (Chapter 16) noted this when he spoke of the inadvisability of the "three day admission for full developmental work up" of the individual child. This will not be productive in terms of identifying lead-attributable toxicity in the individual, nor will it aid in the identification of a paint, fouling of the nest, or an industrial hazard. Whatever the effect of low doses of lead on CNS function, they are more a regulatory, public health and epidemiologic concern than they are clear-cut causes of obvious clinical dysfunction.

Follow Up: Prospective Study and Clinical Problems

One seemingly attractive proposition to aid understanding of the low dose problem would be to initiate a very large, long term prospective study, with high follow-up rates and measurement of CNS function in various ways. In addition to the usual considerations of cost, time and commitment, however, there is the additional difficulty of the altered management such a group of children would receive. Since lead levels would be known, environmental intervention would have to begin at blood leads 30 μg/100 cc or so. Although the behavior of this group would be of interest, there are still many children in the 30 to 60 μg/100 cc range to whom such data would be relatively inapplicable, especially if negative. There is, I believe, a way out of this dilemma, a validated CNS effect marker. Thus I return again to the importance of the work of Dr. Chisolm and others. Another way would be to take children whose performance had been assessed and to look at lead in shed teeth. This is being done with some of the children who participated in the Perinatal Collaborative Project.

Dr. Chisolm presented an atypical case of a child with an initially low blood lead who turned out to be at risk. This case would not have been evaluated or treated properly if rigid application of Center for Disease Control (CDC) guidelines (CDC, 1978) had been used. Although rigid application of any set of guidelines is not recommended, the CDC guidelines for case finding and follow-up will work almost all the time. They do, of course, need a supplemental dose of clinical judgement and curiosity. This case also brings out a phenomenon known to any practicing epidemiologist. There is an inverse relationship between the "interestingness" of a given patient and the likelihood that he will return for routine follow-up. Considerable ingenuity is necessary to find the "interesting" patients, while those for whom everything is going routinely return unfailingly.

Thus, extra follow-up efforts are to be encouraged, for they sometimes produce surprisingly interesting results.

Dust

The issue of finger contamination with lead dust was brought out by Dr. Charney (Chapter 8). There are two parts to this problem. One is that house dust lead does relate to body burden, and the other is that house dust lead is easily recoverable from finger stick samples. This is another reason to screen with FEP or ZPP, because they are unaffected by much contamination.

Nutrition

Dr. Mahaffey's paper (Chapter 7) on the relationship of diet to susceptibility to lead is the best clinical review of a complicated subject that I have seen. It is unusually clear and should be useful to anyone concerned with this important area.

Program Management

Dr. Siker (Chapter 11) brought out the multiple interfaces that exist in any lead program, and emphasized the necessity of program coordination. This very important point was brought up before and needs emphasis again. A prime time for follow-up loss occurs when a family gets passed from one part of a program to another. Effective coordination and communication between the program parts can prevent this. Dr. Siker also mentioned that in many programs, any physician can obtain a blood lead on a child believed to be at risk. Often, however, the public health nurse is the first to identify such a child. If a list of physicians who are willing to order blood leads or protoporphyrins on such children is made available to the nurses, then the value of the blood test can become part of the child's subsequent medical evaluation. Again, this requires coordination, but it has worked well in North Carolina and deserves a trial.

The Laboratory

The laboratory is crucial in any successful program, and Dr. Mitchell showed some of the pitfalls that even experienced laboratories find (Chapter 12). The point here is that quality control, even when it is up to CDC standards, is no assurance of infallibility. There are obvious sources of variability that are beyond the control of the laboratory, i.e. sample gathering and storage, that introduce bias rather than sampling variation, and thus cannot be dealt with by the lab. A partial solution to this problem, again involving program coordination, is to track samples from collection through arrival in the lab. If a record is kept, the "funny" value attributable to 4 hr of sun exposure in a bus station can at least be suspected. The laboratory should have some person to whom to report suspicious values rather than sending them blithely on to the provider or local health department.

Even when everything works well, recall that any screening program, including lead programs, generates about 50% false positive results on the initial round (Rogan and Gladen, 1978). This has to do with test characteristics as determined by the cutoff value for abnormality and the actual prevalence of the sought after condition. Families should be told that a single positive result does not imply disease in the child and that confirmation will be necessary. This will prevent subsequent confusion and anxiety on the part of families and physicians.

Hazard Abatement: Paint and Other Sources

Hazard abatement is another basic necessity of any program. Good training programs are available and those who have attended them have found them very useful. No child should be returned to a leaded environment, and abatement procedures are the only realistic way that this problem can be avoided. The presentation of the unusual hazard abatement problems in the North Carolina battery factory episode points out that innovation is sometimes necessary. The problem there was that the lead dust brought home by the mostly female workers had contaminated the rugs and cars and house dust and could not be gotten rid of by usual means. That episode is one of three reported outbreaks of undue lead absorption in the children of workers where the source was soiled work clothes (Baker et al., 1977; Morbidity and Mortality Weekly Reports, 1977; Dolcourt et al., 1978). It is the only one in which the workers were women, and again points out the necessity of a good occupational history from both parents. Dr. Chisolm pointed out the wide variety of occupations that involve potential exposure to lead. One that he mentioned, ship breaking, also involves exposure to asbestos.

In general, the occupational exposures of parents should be explored and attention paid to other chemicals besides lead. Another type of history that is going to become necessary is an "energy" history. Burning battery cases for hot starter fuel is having a resurgence in North Carolina and perhaps other places as well.

Treatment and the Continuing Paint Problem

Dr. Graef's description of his treatment program (Chapter 16) underlines the fact that treatment is not all that difficult and that consultation and advice are available on a state and sometimes a regional level. The lack of a specialist in lead intoxication is not a reason for ignoring or not seeking out a lead hazard.

Multiple sources of lead for children, i.e., pencils, batteries, work clothes, dustfall, have been mentioned in these papers. Dr. Houk reminded us that the main source of lead is still lead-based paint (Chapter 19). Lead paint poisoning is still a problem, although fewer cases are reported each year. The resultant lack of publicity should not deter further efforts to prevent the disease entirely, since it is one of the few where such efforts undoubtedly pay off.

Summary and a Case Presentation

In summary, there are four parts to lead screening programs: case finding, abatement, laboratory work and treatment. However excellent the individual parts are, they will not work unless coordinated effectively. Children are more susceptible to lead than adults. This is also true of other environmental agents. Thus, occupational exposure histories and education of parents should take place and should not be limited to lead. Finally, research should continue into areas such as the subclinical effects of low lead levels and factors determining susceptibility. However, there is enough knowledge now to prevent the majority of lead-related illness if such knowledge is applied effectively.

Finally, here is a brief case presentation (Osterud et al., 1973). A 27-yr-old male "hippie" presented himself to the emergency room with weakness, leg cramps, tarry stools and abdominal pain. He was given an appointment for gastrointestinal x-rays and sent out. He returned 2 days later, having lost a kilogram of weight, and was sent out again because his x-rays had not yet been done. He returned the next day for continued abdominal pain and vomiting. The medical technologist noted basophilic stippling on the blood smear. The patient was found to be lead intoxicated and was successfully chelated. His plumbism was due to plum wine, homemade in a chipping enamel bathtub. He had drunk 50 gallons of wine (containing about 3.3 mg of lead) over his 5-mo stay at the Green Parrot Goat Farm, a commune of twelve humans, four dogs, four turkeys, two geese, twenty-nine chickens, eleven goats and one parrot. No one else had an elevated blood lead or comparable exposure. The mixed benefits of technologic advance were recognized, and the next year's wine was made in the stainless steel milk cooler.

References

Angle, C.R. and McIntire, M.S. 1964. Lead poisoning during pregnancy. Am J Dis Child 108:451–439.

Baker, E.L., Folland, D.S., Taylor, T.A., Frank, M., Peterson, W., Lovejoy, G., Cox, D. Houseworth, J. and Landrigan, P.J. 1977. Lead poisoning in children of lead workers. Home contamination with industrial dust. N Engl J Med 296:260–261.

Center for Disease Control (CDC) 1978. Preventing Lead Poisoning in Young Children. USDHEW 00-2629. Atlanta.

Chisolm, Jr. J.J. 1978. Fouling one's own nest. Pediatrics 62(4):614–616.

Dine, M.S. 1979. Evaluation of the free erythrocyte protoporphyrin test in a private practice. Pediatrics 65(2):303–306.

Dolcourt, J.L., Hamrick, H.J., O Tuama, L.A., Wooten, J. and Baker, E.L. 1978. Increased lead burden in children of battery workers. Asymptomatic exposure resulting from contaminated work clothing. Pediatrics 62(4):563–566.

Lancranjan, I., Popesca, H.I., Gavenescu, O.,

Klepsch, I. and Serbanescu, M. 1975. Reproductive ability of workmen occupationally exposed to lead. Arch Environ Health 30:396–401.

Morbidity and Mortality Weekly Reports 26:61, 1977. Increased lead absorption in children of lead workers—Vermont.

Needleman, H.L., Gunnoe, C., Leviton, A., Reed, R., Peresie, H., Maher, C. and Barrett, P. 1979. Deficits in psychological and classroom performance of children with elevated dentine lead levels. N Engl J Med 300 (13):689–695.

Nogaki, K. 1958. On the action of lead on the body of lead refinery workers: Particularly conception, pregnancy and parturition in case of females and on vitality of their newborn. Excerpta Med XVIII 4:2176.

Osterud, H.T., Tufts, E. and Holmes, M.F. 1973. Plumbism at the Green Parrot Goat Farm. Clinical Toxicology 6(1):1–7.

Rogan, W.J. and Gladen, B. 1978. Estimating prevalence with the results of a screening test. Am J Epidemiol 107(1):71–78.

22. Discussion

Discussion for Chapters 1-5.

Dr. Goldberg (Chairman): We were fortunate this morning to have Dr. Lin-Fu's comprehensive introduction to this meeting. Emphasis on the lack of knowledge in specific areas substantiates the necessity for increased research activity on toxic effects of lead and an understanding of the disease process. However, adequate information does exist to support the regulation and elimination of lead hazards.

Dr. Lin-Fu pointed out the history and epidemiology of lead poisoning. Most importantly, she demonstrated that lead poisoning is preventable and discussed the implications of not instituting the necessary programs now.

Dr. Hammond reviewed the metabolism and kinetics of lead distribution and compared the biological effects of lead in children and adults. This was complimented by Dr. Goyer's presentation on organ-specific effects and the relationship between dose and response. These presentations were further developed in the experimental studies of neurotoxicity as reviewed by Dr. Reiter. Together, the papers point out the need for caution in comparing the consequences of lead exposure in animal and clinical studies and the importance of careful documentation of exposure and dose. The biological consequences of high dose short-term exposure do appear to be different from those of low dose long-term exposure.

Before opening the general discussion, I shall ask Dr. Chisolm to present some interesting preliminary clinical data.

Chisolm, J.J., Jr.: **Urinary homovanillic acid (HVA). A possible new biochemical marker for lead—preliminary clinical data**

In children, major emphasis today is being placed on the prevention of lead poisoning, particularly its adverse effects on the developing nervous system. This preventive approach is based upon two major considerations; these are the "critical effect" concept of toxicology as applied to heavy metals and the use of biochemical markers to detect lead toxicity at an early and, hopefully, reversible

211

stage. A toxic metal, such as lead, may have adverse effects in several organ systems, the most commonly affected being the nervous system, the erythrocytes and the kidney. According to the "critical effect" concept, these organs may vary in their sensitivity to lead. The "critical effect" is the most sensitive and specific biologic change beyond acceptable physiologic variation which is caused by the metal. This is shown schematically in Figure 1, in which an increasing internal dose or tissue concentration of a metal such as lead is plotted against increasing severity of the metal's effect in various organ systems, here labeled schematically as Effects I, II and III, respectively. In this drawing, Effect I occurs at the lowest internal dose and is by definition the first or "critical effect." At present there is a general consensus that inhibition of heme synthesis in the erythroid cells of the bone marrow is the "critical effect" of lead. In short, the erythroid cells of the bone marrow are the cells most sensitive to lead. Inhibition of δ-aminolevulinic acid dehydratase activity, increase in the urinary excretion of δ-aminolevulinic acid and coproporphyrins and increased concentration of zinc protoporphyrin in erythrocytes are biochemical markers of this effect. These metabolic changes are reversible. These considerations provide the theoretical basis for using FEP and other biochemical indicators of lead's inhibitory metabolic effect on heme synthesis to detect and monitor children overexposed to lead.

To a very large extent, the consensus that the erythroid cells of the bone marrow are the ones most sensitive to lead is based upon the ready availability of established and sensitive biochemical indicators of lead's adverse effects on heme synthesis coupled with the lack of a sensitive biochemical indicator of lead's adverse effects in the nervous system. (It is generally considered that the kidney is relatively resistant to the effects of lead and so might be considered Effect III in Figure 1.) Ellen Silbergeld and I have been most interested in the

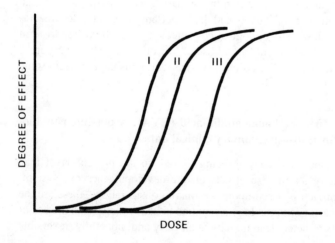

Fig. 1. Schematic diagram of critical effect.

Table 1.   Correlations between blood lead, chelatable lead, urinary lead and various biochemical indicators of adverse metabolic effects.

	PbB	PbU-EDTA	PbU	HVA	ALAU	FEP
Blood lead (PbB)		0.461*	ns	0.729†	0.468*	ns
Chelatable lead (PbU-EDTA)			ns	ns	0.652†	ns
Spontaneous urine lead (PbU)				ns	ns	ns
Homovanillic acid (HVA)					ns	ns
δ-Aminolevulinic acid (ALAU)						ns
"Free" erythrocyte protoporphyrin (FEP)						

* p < .05.
† p < 0.001.

identification of a neurochemical marker for lead. Such a marker would permit comparison of hematopoietic and neurochemical responses to increased lead absorption in individual children. Although experimental studies have demonstrated rather consistently that lead disturbs cholinergic function, no biochemical markers useful in humans are associated with this aspect of lead toxicity. On the other hand, catecholamine neurotransmitters and their catabolites can be measured in blood, urine and CSF in man. For this reason, we chose to look at the catecholamine catabolite, homovanillic acid (HVA), even though experimental studies in rodents have yielded conflicting results regarding lead's effect on catecholamine metabolism and function. In a pilot study, we reported that the levels of homovanillic acid, a major catabolite of dopamine, were elevated in both brain and urine of lead-intoxicated mice and in the urine of six children with blood lead concentrations greater than 60 μg Pb/dl whole blood. The next step in this investigation was to determine whether a dose-response relationship could be demonstrated between lead and the urinary output of HVA in children. I will now summarize the preliminary data so far obtained on this question.

We have now studied 25 asymptomatic children with no record of prior symptoms or therapy for lead poisoning. The children ranged from 19 to 54 mos of age with a median age of 30 mos. Blood lead concentrations ranged from 42 to 72 μg Pb/dl whole blood. Studies were made under controlled dietary and environmental conditions in hospital. FEP and daily outputs of HVA and δ-aminolevulinic acid in urine were measured. After a 4-day control period, all received the calcium disodium EDTA mobilization test. Data were analyzed by least squares linear regression. The statistical analyses are summarized in Table 1. A statistically highly significant relationship was found between blood lead concentration and urinary HVA ($r = 0.729$, $p < 0.001$). Of note is the finding that urinary HVA shows no significant relationship with the heme metabolites such as free erythrocyte protoporphyrin and urinary δ-aminolevulinic acid. Nor is there a significant correlation between HVA and chelatable lead.

The data suggest that the inhibitory effects of lead on heme synthesis are not related to its apparent effect on HVA metabolism. These preliminary findings, if confirmed, may have important clinical implications, for they suggest that one may not be able to predict from lead's effect in one metabolic system, heme synthesis in the erythroid cells of the bone marrow, what its effect may be in another metabolic system such as HVA metabolism. The mechanism by which the urinary excretion of HVA is increased remains to be elucidated. At present, no data in children are available to determine whether these findings represent an effect of lead on the kidney or on catecholamine metabolism in the nervous system.

Table 1 contains another item of clinical importance. No statistically significant relationship was found in this group between FEP and chelatable lead. Taken together, these preliminary data suggest that major emphasis should be placed on serial blood lead measurements in the management of children with increased lead absorption.

Dr. Goldberg: Thank you, Dr. Chisolm, for those illuminating remarks. In his presentation, Dr. Charney carefully reviewed the literature on subencephalo-pathic lead poisoning in children. He pointed out that there are several studies that demonstrate a change of 3 or 4 points in the IQ of young populations. With this as a focal point, I would like to start the discussion with two questions. The first of these is, what are the consequences, both to the individual and society, of a change in IQ of 3 or 4 points; secondly, with the evidence presented both from animal and human studies, can we still argue that we do not have enough data to know that lead is toxic and that intervention is necessary to control and eliminate lead poisoning?

Dr. Charney: Those are provocative questions. I think I took a particularly negative look at the data to try to be as critical as possible. I think it's hard to say what the difference of 3 or 4 IQ points is. I'm not a psychologist and I really don't feel comfortable answering that.

Dr. Pearson: I'm a psychologist. I would say that a change of 3 or 4 IQ points would be deemed significant only if you could show an increase in the distribution of children so affected having IQs in the retarded range of intellectual functioning.

Editor's Note: In what is, perhaps, one of the most comprehensive and critical reviews of the evidence in young children on the significance of asymptomatic increased lead absorption for cognitive and behavioral functioning, Rutter (1980) makes the following comment on the practical implications of a 3 to 5 point reduction in IQ:

"Given that the provisional conclusion on the evidence to date is that it is very likely that psychological impairment occurs in some asymptomatic children with repeated blood lead levels in the 40- to 80-μg/100 ml range, and that it is possible (although much less certain) that impairment sometimes occurs at levels lower than 40, it is necessary to ask what are the practical implications *now?* The cognitive deficits which have been found have usually been of the order of three to five points, and it has been argued that a five-point difference is so trivial in its effects that it can really be ignored. . . That is a totally fallacious argument. It can easily be calculated statistically that a drop of five points in mean IQ (assuming maintenance of the same distribution) for any population must necessarily result in more than a two-fold increase in the percentage of individuals with an IQ below 70, i.e., a *doubling* of the number of mentally retarded children! By no stretch of the imagination could this be regarded as trivial." Rutter, M. 1980. Raised lead levels and impaired cognitive behavioral functioning; A review of the evidence. Develop Med Child Neurol 22: Suppl. 1.

Dr. Graef: At what point can we extrapolate from experimental animal data to human exposures, if at all, in terms of perinatal versus slightly later exposures to lead (i.e., the 1- to 2-yr-old child)?

Dr. Reiter: That's a good question: I'm afraid that I can't answer it, because the data are just not there. There are relatively few studies which have attempted to look at critical periods of exposure. As you know, the developmental time course in the human and in the rat are quite different. I don't think that researchers have taken enough time to examine what these critical periods are and how they correlate with the human. The nonspecificity of lead in terms of producing neurotoxicity is such that the effect would depend to a large extent on the period in which the animal was exposed simply because, if you're producing the nonspecific damage to developing neurons and these neurons have presumably different functions, then the effects that you're going to see are going to be highly dependent on this exposure. What needs to be done is to look more carefully at how lead affects these maturational processes. One arbitrary period and system should be studied; if we can make some generalities about how lead disrupts these systems, then we should have some ability to predict what would happen in the clinical situation when exposures are performed during different periods in which we know the developmental time course of the brain.

Dr. Mahaffey: I have a question for Dr. Reiter on the data he showed on lead and calcium interacting in the nervous system. Is there any indication that variation in dietary calcium produces much effect on the concentration of calcium in CNS?

Dr. Reiter: Lead and calcium interact at many levels, including absorption from the gut. In most of these animal studies, there has been little attempt to control calcium levels in the diet. Since these effects have been demonstrated in vitro, as well as in vivo, it seems to me that it's a fairly robust effect of lead; if anything, it would be a compounding factor in the in vivo studies.

Dr. Mahaffey: I was thinking that we assume that, with a functioning parathyroid gland and adequate levels of Vitamin D intake, the bone is such a reservoir of calcium that you wouldn't expect too much difference in calcium concentration; I thought that perhaps as a pharmacologist you were aware of relevant data.

Dr. Hammond: I was very interested in Dr. Chisolm's data showing no correlation between HVA and FEP. It brought to mind a study which we recently completed regarding lead exposure in smelter workers. First, it is not only children who seem to have some neurological effects, that is, central effects, it also appears to be adults. The evidence is not so solid and perhaps the exposure conditions are considerably higher, but there was a high correlation in adults between positive response to a symptom questionnaire relating to the brain, trouble falling asleep and trouble calculating, on the one hand, and not only the blood lead, but also ALA, both in the plasma and in the urine, but not the FEP. Do the intermediates of heme synthesis which accumulate in the course of lead exposure in fact contribute to the neurological effects? In porphyria, there is sometimes suspicion that some of the central nervous system effects of porphyria may be associated with accumulation of heme intermediates.

Dr. Chisolm: There also are some suggestive but far from conclusive experimental data indicating that ALA may be a putative neurotransmitter. Specifically, its molecular structure resembles that of γ-aminobutyric acid (GABA). The hypothesis that ALA may interfere with GABA function is still being tested.

In both severe, acute lead poisoning and acute intermittent porphyria, which share similarities in their clinical symptomology, the levels of ALA in both plasma and urine are comparably and highly elevated; i.e., 50- to 100-fold above the normal range. None of the other metabolites in the heme biosynthetic pathway have been linked to the neurological manifestations of either plumbism or acute intermittent porphyria. Administration of heme to patients with severe acute porphyria both suppresses heme synthesis (as anticipated) with lowering of ALA and porphobilinogen levels and is associated with marked reduction in clinical symptoms. These dramatic clinical studies give credence to the hypothesis that accumulation of excess heme metabolites, particularly ALA, are causally related to the acute neurological manifestations of porphyria.

In the group of children upon which I have just reported, most were completely asymptomatic in the clinical sense and ALA and HVA levels in urine were modestly to moderately elevated. The ALA levels in these children did not approach the levels seen in acute lead encephalopathy. What is interesting about these data is the observation that some children showed elevated ALA, but not HVA, while in others urinary HVA was elevated, but urinary ALA was not. This suggests that various metabolic pathways affected by lead may not necessarily respond in a uniform pattern; rather, the relative responses of pathways may vary between children.

Dr. Reiter: I'd like to expand on that a bit. The increased excretion of metabolites is probably related to an effect which is ongoing; the morphological changes associated with exposure during early development, at least in animals, are going to be permanent alterations. They are probably not going to be associated with these types of biochemical alterations. I would hate to see that used as an index of poisoning, because you may have missed the period of exposure which is producing the effect, and you may still have altered CNS function, but you would not be able to demonstrate it by the metabolites.

Dr. Chisolm: First, I think Dr. Reiter made it quite clear in his formal presentation that lead has a multiplicity of toxic effects in the developing nervous system. The effects of lead on catecholamine metabolism is but one of these effects and not necessarily the most serious. At present, we are dependent in the clinical field on batteries of neuropsychological tests for evaluation of the impact of lead on the nervous system. These tests are nonspecific and often global in their scope. It would be most helpful to identify some relatively specific biochemical indicator of the effect of lead on metabolism in the nervous system. HVA may possibly be such an indicator. It may not be the best, but it is a beginning.

Dr. Mushak: I have two general questions for Drs. Goyer and Hammond. First, are there thresholds for the various effects of lead such as its effects on hematopoietic tissue? Second, when does a biochemical perturbation become an adverse health effect?

Dr. Goyer: Let me make a quick response. By threshold, I guess you mean a level of lead below which there is no effect? This has to do with the tools that we have to measure; we're much better at measuring biochemical things than clinical ones. In terms of when that becomes an adverse health effect, for heme products, increased presence of heme products, excretion in the urine or elevation in blood, I don't think that there's any evidence that these are toxic in any way. Very high levels of ALA may be the exception, as we have just heard.

Dr. Hammond: I would like to make two comments. First, on the use of the word threshold, that is a very nebulous concept. If you had a group of ten rats and you had five doses of a poison, 1, 10, 50, 100 and 1000 mg, and you gave those doses to groups of ten rats, you might find that the threshold is 10 mg/k. Now, if you increase the size of the group to 100 rats per group, the threshold would go down, because the larger the population that you study, the lower the threshold, because of the increased probability of finding the unusually sensitive. This is the difficulty with that term threshold. It's much more meaningful to talk in terms of probability of occurrence versus dose. For example, if you're talking about cancer, the acceptable level of risk at least for the EPA is something on the order of 1 in 100,000. The threshold that you get is usually not even experimentally verifiable; it's extrapolated. I think we have to think of that concept in regard to any poison, including lead. The other point is the one that Dr. Goyer made about the implications of some of these sub-clinical perturbations and heme synthesis. Obviously, the system is compensated when a rise in protoporphyrin occurs at a blood level of 25 or 30, because there is no decrement in hemoglobin. The real concern is whether such an individual who is challenged with some other insult to his hematopoietic system might not show an additive effect. There has only been one experiment in which dogs were exposed to levels of lead which did not cause a decrement in hemoglobin, but only a moderate rise in ALA in the urine. That group of dogs and a control group were then bled down to 50% of original blood volume and the rate of return of the hematocrit of hemoglobin to normal was measured. In this particular experiment, there was no difference between the two groups in that respect. Unfortunately, the level of ALA excretion which was enhanced by the lead exposure was very modest. I don't think that is a final answer; rather, it is an example of the kind of approach which should be used in trying to establish the meaning of sub-clinical effects which is to seek out the most logical covariants which might add width to the lead effect to produce an otherwise unobservable clinical response.

Discussion for Chapters 6-10.

Dr. Rogan: One thing you didn't talk about in terms of nutrition and absorption of lead is lead in food. Is there much of lead in food, particularly in things like infant formula?

Dr. Mahaffey: The amount of lead in infant formula has dropped dramatically over the past 7 years. The levels are now measured in parts per billion, which is very low as far as the concentration goes. However, remember the volume of formula that infants consume; it can be as much as a liter or 1500 ml of formula per day. This is particularly important with the trend to keeping infants on formula alone until they're perhaps 6 mos of age, which is something that many pediatricians now recommend. Various types of formulas are marketed. There are condensed, ready to feed and dried formulas, different ones will contain different amounts of lead. Probably the best choice is using dried formula and reconstituting it with water. There again it becomes complicated, because it depends on the water supply. We also have the unfortunate case of tea kettles that are used to boil water that have been soldered with lead. We think we have those off the market. It's hard to answer general questions, but certainly the amount of lead in infant formulas has declined. We find that many infants have "normal" blood leads, certainly under 20 μg/dl. In rural areas, if you survey 100 infants, you will find that around 80 of them have a blood lead under 10 μg/dl. It is not an overwhelming source of lead. The infant formulas are highly important in that they are nutritionally balanced. They are good sources of iron, good sources of calcium, and in some cases the zinc level in these formulas has been raised. So you really have to say that they do substantially more good than anything else. There has, in fact, been an active program to get the lead in foods lowered and it has been successful. As an aside, we used to see infant juices marketed in cans, but at this point, they are marketed in glass bottles; this has markedly reduced the lead content of these juices (and formulas). We are not sure they are as low as they can get, partly because we must distinguish between the amount of lead that's present in the background, the soil, the air and the water that are present when the food is grown, and the amount added during processing. However, we do know that the levels are lower.

Dr. Mitchell: The problem in the lead poisoning field seems to be to make a modest improvement in a very large number of children. Wouldn't you expect that the most effective thing we could do would be routine but fairly modest multi-mineral supplementation for the kids that turn up with moderately elevated lead levels?

Dr. Mahaffey: I think it certainly could do much good. With mineral supplements, going from deficient to normal levels is important. There is a very real area known as mineral toxicity, we don't exactly know where it begins. If you are working at 50% above recommended levels, you may be alright, but don't try adding ten times the recommended amount of mineral supplements. Also, it seems that iron and calcium effects apply to cadmium as well as to lead. Diet is important in protecting against a number of environmental hazards.

Dr. Lynam: Dr. Mahaffey, you point out the importance of nutrition in lead absorption, with poor nutrition, low iron, increased lead absorption. Poor nutrition, especially low iron, has also been associated with effects such as decreased performance in IQ tests. I think Dr. Oski has reported such results. The same type of deficit is attributed to lead. I wonder if poor nutrition might not be the cause of the poor performance and increased lead is associated.

Dr. Mahaffey: Certainly in the animal experimental data, there can be very real confounding effects of nutrition on the results, particularly in cases where you have animals that are treated with lead, whose body weight is only 50 to 60% of the control animals that weren't treated with lead. There you may have very real nutrition interactions. There certainly is evidence for behavioral effects and effects on learning and on brain development of severe undernutrition in humans. But with probably very few exceptions, you don't see that degree of undernutrition in the lead-exposed subjects, because for the most part, these studies have investigated relatively healthy individuals. Also, if you have changes in nutritional status, you automatically have a confounding effect on the amount of lead that is absorbed. You can have a confounding of the distribution of lead. It can be involved, but you certainly can't attribute all the effects that have been shown in human studies of moderate levels of lead exposure to nutrition.

Dr. Goldberg: Dr. Cataldo, the data presented earlier by Dr. Hammond (Chapter 6) strongly suggest that pica for lead occurs only episodically, perhaps once per week. My first question then is, how effective will behavior modification procedures be in controlling an infrequent episodic activity?

Dr. Cataldo: Behavior modification is based on the experimentally documented principle that behavior is (at least in part) a function of its consequences. Thus, the frequency of a behavior, like pica, will decrease if consequences are changed from those which maintain the rate to those which decelerate the rate. *Rapid* behavior change is a function of the effectiveness of the consequences chosen, the consistency with which the prescribed program is carried out and the number of opportunities (behavior rate) to which consequences can be applied. The power of chosen consequences to change behavior being equal, behaviors which occur infrequently will take longer to modify if for no other reason than there are less opportunities to apply consequences per unit of time (days, weeks, months). In addition, from a practical standpoint, it is often difficult for parents to consistently employ a behavior change program if the behavior occurs infrequently. Therefore, decreasing all pica might be preferable to a program which only focuses on eliminating consumption of lead containing materials. However, regardless of the predictions about modifying a low frequency behavior with a parental intervention, behavior modification may offer a clinically relevant addition to lead poisoning prevention programs. Considering the alternatives the public health and scientific communities have been able to offer to date and the lack of risks of behavior modification procedures, a small scale extension of our pilot demonstration to determine clinical benefit for children in daily living environments seems a reasonable course to pursue.

Dr. Goldberg: Dr. Charney has pointed out that household dust lead and the amount of lead on a child's hands are closely correlated and that the hand lead is one of the best, if not the best, predictor of blood lead concentration in children. It was Donald Barltrop, I believe, who pointed out that over 50% of young children engage in repetitive daily hand to mouth activity. Your presentation suggested that behavioral modification, to be effective, requires an intensive, one-on-one therapeutic program. How effective will this be in the public health setting in the presence of significant environmental lead pollution? Generally, those public health measures that have been most effective have been simple and have involved modification of the environment rather than modification of human behavior.

Dr. Cataldo: Our pilot studies of children in hospital settings show that hand-to-mouth activity can be successfully modified and that as the rate decreases less one-to-one contact is necessary. But, as you point out, one-to-one contact is necessary to provide consequences for behavior. If by a public health setting you mean the home and community environment of the child, then there is no inherent reason why behavior modification procedures as we suggest for pica and mouthing would not be effective as similar procedures have been for many other behaviors occurring in the community and home. Public health procedures which eliminate a health risk by eliminating the cause of the problem are indeed often simple and the solution of choice. The problem, of course, is that we can not always modify the physical environment sufficiently to remove the cause of a health problem. My knowledge of the literature on the lead problem and the proceedings of this conference certainly indicate that removing or sufficiently reducing lead in all environments is not now feasible. Perhaps until the lead environmental hazard is eliminated, the science of the experimental analysis of behavior, to which I refer in my paper, can be added to the procedures currently employed in order to further reduce lead absorption in children. However, let me say very clearly here, that regardless of successful behavior modification approaches to pica and mouthing, now and in the future, such data should never be considered a justification for not eliminating dangerous levels of lead in children's environments. Behavior modification approaches to reduce lead ingestion could never be as successful nor appropriate a solution as reducing lead in the environment below dangerous levels.

Dr. Mitchell: What is the single most important thing that would be effective in reducing treatment costs and the medical sequellae?

Mr. O'Hara: Certainly coordinating the medical and environmental treatment efforts. The treatment of children is in some ways more difficult than the treatment of adult lead workers. Whereas the lead worker may be removed from his exposure, his place of employment, and treated with relative safety at home, the child cannot be treated at home without serious risk since the child's principal sources of exposure are usually in his home.

Discussion for Chapters 11-18.

Dr. Mahaffey: I understand that the x-ray fluorometers used by housing examiners in testing for the presence of leaded paint are not sensitive to low levels of lead in paint. While these instruments may be important in getting a court order to do something about housing, I believe their sensitivity level still leaves a fairly high amount of lead untested insofar as toxic exposures are concerned. Experimental data from human adult volunteers ingesting about 1000 μg/day show that they begin to get hematologic changes in 14 days.

Dr. Chadzynski: The x-ray fluoresence analyzer is the most suitable means the public health worker has for making a large number of measurements quickly. It is true that the minimum detectable level, 0.7 mg/sq cm, is much higher than the detection limits for the more sensitive but time consuming chemical methods, which can measure amounts of lead as low as 0.06 mg/gram of paint or less.

Dr. Mahaffey: Is there much lead in currently available putty, plaster and caulking compounds? The older literature suggests that there may be.

Mr. Sobolesky: We have never found much lead in plaster in the interior of homes in Philadelphia. This may be due to the fact that Philadelphians have rarely painted plaster with lead-containing paints. However, lead paints have apparently been applied over plaster for a number of years in many other cities. Lead has a tendency to leech into plaster because of its porosity, so I am certain that you will find lead in plaster if lead paint has been applied in the past. Plaster, itself, does not contain lead. We have not found lead in putty. However, we do find lead paints applied over putty. Finally, I must make a comment as far as occupational exposure is concerned. There is one occupation that we in Philadelphia have just identified as a potential problem both in the worker and their children. That occupation is ballistics testing and target practice by police officers. This has, of course, been reported in the occupational and environmental literature, but I doubt that you find much about it in the pediatric journals.

Ms. Erman: In Washington, D.C., homeowners are responsible for abatement of lead hazards in their homes. Can the people who have experience with abatement give any suggestions to parents who are responsible for abating lead hazards in their own homes? I am particularly interested in those that are safest and easiest.

Mr. Sobolesky: In our program in Philadelphia, we do have a specification sheet that goes with every order to a property owner. This outlines the procedures to follow, the use of respirators, the requirement that the owner not repaint until we reinspect to see that all lead-based paint is taken off down to the bare wood. There are, of course, OSHA regulations that apply to the removal of lead-based paint; however, these regulations are not too specific, because OSHA has not recognized lead-based paint removal as an occupational hazard. In Philadelphia, HUD contracts with private contractors to remove lead-based paint, but they give no instructions and they do not monitor the workers. I feel certain that blood lead levels in these workers rise; however, no one appears to be paying any attention to this fact. We have called attention to this point to these contractors many, many times. The same thing occurs in sandblasting operations. HUD tried at one time to use sandblasting in homes. During sandblasting operation in a confined space, you would not be able to see the worker after even a few minutes. Under these conditions, the worker needs a forced air respirator from an outside source. Unfortunately, the windows are often blown out and much of the woodwork is chewed up. We would certainly like to see this aspect of occupational lead exposure improved.

Dr. Houk: I'd like to make a comment on the question of finances. If a child is identified as part of the Federally funded childhood lead poisoning project, it is required that the project provide abatement methodology for the financially unable owner/occupant to abate lead hazards in his/her own house. If the owner/occupant is not financially able and is making enough money to pay Federal income tax, the removal of lead-based paint from inside and around the house is deductible as a medical expense from one's personal Federal income tax, provided that the abatement has been ordered by a physician.

Dr. Dolcourt: I have two questions for Dr. Chisolm. How do you handle a child with increased lead burden at the time of intercurrent stresses such as infections. Will such stresses mobilize lead from bone and so increase the blood lead level and associated risk due to lead? My second question relates to pregnancy. We in North Carolina have encountered some pregnant working women with elevated blood lead levels due to occupational exposure. I wonder if you have any thoughts about whether an increased maternal lead burden may endanger fetuses during future pregnancies.

Dr. Chisolm: With regard to your first question, I believe the thought that infection may mobilize significant amounts of lead from bone dates back to clinical reports in the 1930's. These clinical reports do not separate the role of possible mobilization of lead from bone and continued excessive oral intake of lead. I, personally, have encountered only rare instances during the 1950's in some patients in hospitals convalescing from acute encephalopathy in whom mobilization of lead from bone may have occurred. I refer to a few observations in which no clinical symptoms occurred, but chelatable lead and urinary coproporphyrin did increase markedly during infection in patients hospitalized over a 1- to 3-mo period. I am speaking here of patients whose initial blood lead concentrations fell within the range of 200 to 800 μg/dl whole blood. More recently, we have not seen any evidence of exacerbation of lead toxicity during current infections in patients with PbB in the range of 50 to 80 μg/dl hospitalized at Mt. Washington.

The question of increased lead absorption in the fetus is indeed a difficult one to answer insofar as present day conditions are concerned. On the basis of data obtained in occupationally exposed women during the 19th century, a British commission recommended in about 1910 that women should not be employed in the lead trades. They based this recommendation on clinical reports, which indicated that the rates of spontaneous abortions and stillbirths were increased in women with symptomatic plumbism. In retrospect, we can estimate that such women were probably carrying blood lead concentrations in the range of 100 to 200 μg/dl whole blood. This, we hope, does not occur under modern day industrial hygiene practices. We have, however, no data upon which to estimate risk associated with a modest increase in lead absorption during pregnancy. However, experimental data show that lead freely crosses the placenta and causes adverse effects in the offspring at rather low doses of lead. At birth, maternal and cord blood lead concentrations in humans are equivalent. As for the question of mobilization of lead from bone during future pregnancies, nothing is known.

Dr. Graef: Dr. Chisolm, occasionally I have been asked to see a child who is scheduled for elective surgery and who has an elevated blood lead level. The question arises as to whether such children are normal candidates for general anesthesia. When the surgery is elective, we have generally opted to deal with the lead problem first and lower the blood lead levels prior to elective surgery. On the other hand, I know of no clinical data that would suggest that elevation in blood lead concentration increases operative risk. Do you have any comment on this point?

Dr. Chisolm: No, I use the same approach. I would like to see the blood lead concentration less than 50 μg/dl before elective surgery is undertaken.

Dr. Hammond: I am a bit unclear as to the role of the provocative EDTA mobilization test in clinical diagnosis. It seems to me that there is a very good correlation between blood lead and PbU-EDTA both in adults and in children regardless of whether the elevated blood lead concentration is due to current exposure or excess exposure in the remote past. Since Dr. Chisolm is the one who has provided this information as it relates to children, I would like to hear his comment on the role of the EDTA mobilization test.

Dr. Chisolm: I do not use this test in the practical day-to-day management of children with elevated blood lead concentrations. I feel that one can get enough information from a thorough environmental history, the medical history of the child and serial blood lead concentrations to make a decision concerning treatment. I feel that the EDTA mobilization test is quite useful within the context of clinical research. Practically, the test is limited because of the difficulty in getting complete urine collections from young children. Since a single intramuscular injection of the drug does not produce a uniform diuresis throughout either an 8-hr or 24-hr period, one can be grossly misled if, for example, the specimen representing the peak diuresis of lead is lost. Such factors as the estimated duration of excess exposure and the age of the child play an important role in therapeutic decisions in chronic cases; trends in PbB and FEP, as I have tried to illustrate, can also play an important part in therapeutic decisions.

Dr. Graef: I'm not certain that there's a great deal of disagreement between Dr. Chisolm and myself. It is probably true that we do EDTA mobilization tests many times when we really do not have to, as it often confirms what we already know about the child. However, I think that there are a number of borderline situations in which the lead mobilization test does add an important piece of information about a clinical decision on whether or not to give an individual child chelation therapy. It is also my opinion that the EDTA mobilization test may be particularly useful in chronic cases where one is deciding whether a second, third or fourth course of chelation therapy would be effective in mobilizing a significant amount of the body lead burden into the urine.

Index